SACRED
REVOLUTION

*A Woman's path to Love,
Power & Sensual Enlightenment*

VANYA SILVERTEN

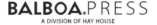
BALBOA.PRESS
A DIVISION OF HAY HOUSE

Balboa Press books may be ordered through booksellers or by contacting:

Balboa Press
A Division of Hay House
1663 Liberty Drive
Bloomington, IN 47403
www.balboapress.com
1 (877) 407-4847

Because of the dynamic nature of the Internet, any web addresses or links contained in this book may have changed since publication and may no longer be valid. The views expressed in this work are solely those of the author and do not necessarily reflect the views of the publisher, and the publisher hereby disclaims any responsibility for them.

The author of this book does not dispense medical advice or prescribe the use of any technique as a form of treatment for physical, emotional, or medical problems without the advice of a physician, either directly or indirectly. The intent of the author is only to offer information of a general nature to help you in your quest for emotional and spiritual well-being. In the event you use any of the information in this book for yourself, which is your constitutional right, the author and the publisher assume no responsibility for your actions.

Any people depicted in stock imagery provided by Getty Images are models, and such images are being used for illustrative purposes only. Certain stock imagery © Getty Images.

Print information available on the last page.

ISBN: 978-1-9822-4350-0 (sc)
ISBN: 978-1-9822-4352-4 (hc)
ISBN: 978-1-9822-4351-7 (e)

Library of Congress Control Number: 2020903238

Balboa Press rev. date: 03/19/2020

Contents

For my daughter:
Aurora Elektra

Some people reach for stars,
Other's birth galaxies.
As a woman you get to do both.

Prologue

Long before organized religion, humanity was centered around nature worship. Spiritual communion was exchanged between trees, animals, the earth, the sky, the stars, and the moon. Life revolved around honoring the seasonal changes and observing the signs sent by life itself to ensure survival. Women, as the bearers of life, had a greater connection to the mysteries of the universe. They discovered that their menstrual cycle had a rhythm just like the seasons and the moon; their bodies waxed into creating life at ovulation and waned into the depths of their soul at menstruation. This process, month after month, brought much awareness and many insights to both the seen and unseen worlds. Their intuitive and psychic senses developed because they learned to translate the finer energy vibrations that rippled through the fabric of life.

Women discovered that family members who had passed over still existed and brought guidance and assistance. They learned to communicate with trees and thus discovered the healing properties of herbs and flowers. These women could feel the stars calling and guiding them. They befriended the moon, discovered the monthly tides of their emotions, and understood the reasons they felt so deeply. They taught their daughters these ways so they could deepen the practice and have greater communion with all that exists.

Each generation continued to teach their daughters about the sacred and intuitive connection to life, and each generation refined it until it became known as secret women's business. This secret woman's business provided a map and a manual to interpret and navigate through life.

It explained the subtle phenomenon that occurred in nature when a decision had to be made. Women learned to read when the sun fell on their face as a sign to move forward, and if the wind blew, it was a sign to stop and reconsider. As their awareness of subtle life frequencies increased, their communion to nature deepened. The great nature Goddess was born, and many ceremonies were made to honor the sacred connection a woman had to life.

This sacred and psychic connection with nature and the universe was a full-body experience. The vibrations of guidance rippled through women's thoughts, blossomed in their hearts, electrified their skin, rang through their bones, and danced through their muscles. This intuitive connection to life was a sensual delight—women could smell, hear, touch, see, and taste the vibrations flowing through the universe. Every wave of information they encountered offered wisdom and insight into the mechanics of life. Women become wiser every time they opened themselves to receive guidance. Their communion was so profound that a love affair with life developed.

An energetic union took place between a woman's body and the vibrations that emitted from every living thing. Her beautiful body temple became a conduit to translate the frequencies being sent to her. The higher the vibrations received, the more orgasmic the sensations were felt. An orgasm was not a localized experience—it was an all-body, all-spirit experience that awakened the vibrations of love existing in her cells to be released. Her unique vibration of love was activated to radiate and bless life. The unique vibration of love she felt shining from every cell of her body was her soul. When she felt her soul, she felt alive, full and complete. Any sense of loneliness or isolation evaporated because she had union with her most compatible soul mate: the entire universe.

The more a woman opened her body temple to the universe, the more she felt life making love to her, and the more she felt herself. Each orgasm of life that passed through her brought an awareness that strengthened her core, gave her a glow, and made her feel beautiful. Each one made her feel more like herself. Her uniqueness was revealed every time her body breathed in the universe, because it gave her the energy to exhale more of herself back into life.

This movement became her path of sensual enlightenment, and the pleasure of this path called her to refine her senses so she could tune into the finer, more subtle frequencies of love that the universe offered. These delicate vibrations gave her the most luxurious pleasure sensations, enabling her to birth her beauty, her divine femininity, her goddess self, into life. The journey into love was not always easy, but the promise of a more sublime experience made it compelling. She became a huntress of love. She discovered how her inner awareness could refine her body temple to transduce, the beautiful frequencies emitted from the universe. She stripped her ego and opened her being, so that these pulses of love could be felt everywhere. Through this, she discovered the divine universe of love was a realm of reality, and she learned to ensure its existence.

She allowed herself to ride the waves of love's ecstasy and so discovered the dynamic intelligence love provided. She could be seen running naked through the fields, frolicking in the waters, and basking on the rocks with her legs parted so the divine universe could enter and touch her depths. Through this process, she returned to her original essence; she came home to her origin and became one with love. She married the divine universe, vowing to uphold love because love was the most exquisite reality that existed.

"Love is the most exquisite reality that exists."

Through this union many initiations were created to honor the path of love. Many fertility ceremonies were performed so love could be a bridge to life. They would connect to the divine universe, and through intentions and prayers, they wove love into their families, into their tribe, and into the land. Woman's connection to love opened her heart, and she felt a deep compassion for all of creation. She was in love with life, and she desired to return everything that was not in alignment to love back to love. She learned that through compassion everything could heal, and so through the generations, the gift of healing was cultivated.

The gift of healing came first as the ability to transmit the vibration of love, from the heavens through the body, and into the patient. The vibrations of love had a natural intelligence. They could unlock and transmute the harmful frequencies causing sickness in the body. By observing the healing power of love, these women eventually were able to translate what the divine universe wanted to communicate to the listener. They voiced messages, warnings, and solutions, and the oracle was born. As a woman's connection to the divine universe increased, so did her ability to transform the life around her. For some, this ability made them priestesses; for others, it made them great mothers. Both paths made women the keepers and creators of love.

Every girl, before she became a mother, was taught to choose a man with a loving heart, and she was also taught the ways to birth her man into love through sexual intimacy. Her body, when honored and respected through lovemaking, opened like a flower, blossomed with love, and excreted a nectar from her body. Her juices were an elixir coded with the intelligence of the divine universe. The more her partner made love to her, the more her body became a blessing for him. When he entered her, he fell into heaven, and she would wrap the divine universe around him with her arms and legs. Into each other they would melt; into each other they would dissolve; into each other they would disappear. Together they became the vibration of love. It was only when her partner journeyed with her into love that she would allow a sacred conception to occur.

Through a divine orgasm, she would open her body to be a vessel and welcome a spark of love into her womb. In her next heavenly orgasm, she would pull the divine universe into her sacred womb and infuse her baby to be formed with love. Throughout her pregnancy she ensured that her body remained connected to the divine universe. In this way she surrounded herself with the dimension of love, so that when she gave birth, her baby was born into love. Throughout her child's life, she would weave the wisdom, power, and beauty of love into his or her being. She would teach her child ways to contact this energy. The more she taught love, the more she embodied it. The gift of love was thus transmitted through the generations.

The greatest gift love taught these women was self-love. They were taught from an early age that love was their superpower and that no one, no matter how horrible or abusive, could ever destroy it. These women were taught to cultivate the love they had for themselves. They were taught by their mothers to become their own best friend and soul mate. They learned to travel deep into their body and meet the vibration of the divine universe that existed in each of their cells. The love they had for themselves became the fuel to help them travel deeper and deeper into their inner worlds. The more they loved themselves, the more they could love the divine universe that existed within them. The more they loved themselves, the more their inner beauty became their outer radiance. These women glowed, and their presence blessed life because everywhere they went, so did heaven. The more they loved themselves, the more they expressed their unique vibration of love.

Just as a symphony is an elaborate orchestra of sound, so too is love. Every woman who allowed love to pass through her, also allowed love to filter through her uniqueness. Love, then, was able to emanate through her body as a unique vibration. Every time a woman allowed love to pass though her, she was able to feel the truth of herself. Every time she loved herself, she felt loved by the divine universe. The cycle of love continued until she could uphold the greatest vow: "know thyself." To "know thyself" meant she could master love in every situation; she could uphold the wisdom of love and heal that which was out of alignment to love. It meant that she had a voice; her words had power and she was unafraid to speak. Knowing herself meant she was able to stand strong in her power. No person, no lover or situation could ever cause her to waiver. Love made her strong to her core—because love was her core.

'Love makes you strong to the core because it is your core.'

Just like everyone else, she endured heartbreak, loss, sickness, grief and stress but no life situation, no matter how terrifying could ever break her. She knew that whatever happened, she had the ability to die and rebirth herself. Throughout her life she did this a million times. She let go of what no longer worked and reclaimed what did; she did this until her version of heaven was created in reality. She learned that every time love broke in her life, it was the divine universe saying there was a more exquisite experience of love available. All she had to do was expand her unique vibration of love through her body and use it to call the greater wisdom of love to guide her.

She belonged to no one other than the love that pulsed through her cells and the love that shimmered around her. She may have been married; she may have committed her life to her family—but she could never be owned, controlled, dominated, or abused. She belonged to love. This may have frustrated others, and at times she may have been called selfish and crazy, but none of this mattered because the path of love was too delicious. Through the trials and tribulations of life, she may have veered of track at times or collapsed into heartbreak, forgetting the great healing wisdom that lived inside her and all around her. Sometimes the disconnect might have lasted for days, months, or even years, but as soon she chose not to be a victim, she remembered the path of love and found her way back to origin.

The path of love was not always an easy one. It required her to speak up, at times rejecting family obligations, cultural requirements, and collective conditioning. Her perceived rebellion, her "wild," rule-breaking behavior brought her a liberation and a freedom to venture deeper into love. The more her heart broke, the more rules she broke in order to return to the truth of love. This process brought much clarity about the mechanics of life, and the more clarity she gained, the more she was able to heal life and return it to love. Love was her greatest friend, her dearest teacher, and her most cosmic lover. She fell in love with LOVE.

The more she fell in love with love, the more she fell in love with herself, and the more she was able to love life. She had a love affair with the divine universe—she romanced all that existed. Her journey to oneness was a path of sensual enlightenment.

The story of these ancient women lives inside of you. Somewhere in the distant past of your DNA is their loving intelligence. It shines through your cells, warms your body, and desires to radiate out into life so that you, too, can experience sensual enlightenment and revolutionize your life.

Are you ready to remember that which you already are?

Introduction

When I was thirty-four years old, I had an awakening that changed my life forever. I discovered that my sensuality was a path toward enlightenment and my body was a vehicle to embody heaven. It was *the* awakening I had longed for. For years I searched for it in relationships; I tried to find it through self-healing and by voraciously reading spiritual books, but I didn't experience the transformation and insight that I was seeking.

You see, I've always been spiritual, even as a child growing up in Australia. Deep inside I felt a light that wanted to burst out and shine through me. But I was so cluttered with limiting beliefs and lower emotions that my beauty was caged up inside, unable to escape. I desperately wanted to radiate this light into the world so I could feel alive, vibrant, and connected to life.

Unfortunately, my childhood, which was filled with a lot of dysfunction, kept my beauty and light from emerging. My parents frequently divorced and remarried different people. I grew up in eight separate families, all with different stepparents and step-siblings. My family, whatever it consisted of at the moment, moved every six months, forcing me to go to ten different schools. Life was chaotic and unpredictable, making me feel very confused and abandoned.

My best childhood memories were living in the Daintree Rainforest on the northeast coast of Queensland, when I was about nine years old. Our house was so isolated, that the only way to get to it was via a small boat in a crocodile-infested river. I remember my younger brother and I waking up to the sounds of chirping birds, running naked through the forest, surrounded by clearwater creeks, majestic trees, and exotic animals. We were homeschooled, and I communicated with our teacher and the other students via two-way radio. This was the happiest period for me where I felt nature was growing me up instead of my crazy family, but it didn't last long. Just as we settled in, off we went to the next home, the next family dynamic, and the next school.

By the time I was a teenager, I had developed severe anxiety and an eating disorder that caused me to spiral into a vortex of self-hatred. Given the instability of my childhood, I felt extremely troubled about my life and my future. But that light was still shining within me amid all the chaos, willing me to keep moving forward. When I was twenty-one, I packed my bags and bought a one-way ticket for London to begin a new life.

My Spiritual Journey

One of the many hurdles I faced in England was my belief in fairy tales (rather than in my own abilities and feminine strength). I harbored the romantic illusion that the only way my light could be freed was by finding Prince Charming. Yet after a myriad failed relationships, I was still searching to be "completed" and loved into wholeness. I later discovered that my relationships never worked out because I attracted people who were dysfunctional, just as my family had been, and this only left me feeling more heartbroken.

Then one day, I decided to embark on a journey of self healing. I knew if I did not, I would repeat the dysfunctional patterns of my family. After sending a request to the universe to find me the right modality, Theta Healing® crossed my path, and I discovered a technique that easily helped me to heal and recover my sense of self until I felt empowered. It taught me to reprogram my family patterning, transformed my limited beliefs, awakened my intuitive and healing abilities, and most importantly reconnected me back to love. Theta Healing® helped me so much that I studied and trained to become a Master Theta Healing® Practitioner and Teacher. Since then, I've worked with more than 10,000 students and clients from over fifty countries, the majority of whom have been women. Most of my clients come to me with eating disorders, body-image issues, lack of self-esteem, heartbreak, an inability to attract and maintain healthy relationships, spiritual confusion, female health problems, and a need to believe in themselves. All of them, like me—and, I'm guessing, like you—wanted to feel loved and learn how to have the confidence to live their best life. Although I helped them heal and return to a greater understanding of love and self love, I did not realise the essential missing ingredient until I was thirty-four years old.

My Sensual Awakening

It was my Grandmother's eightieth birthday that called me back home to Australia. While I was there, I visited the Daintree Rainforest where I had once felt so happy and free. It is a prehistoric forest, with no electricity and few human inhabitants. Nature there has run wild for a millennia. As soon as I entered the rainforest the energy of earth rose up through my feet, legs, hips, and activated my sexual energy. My womb space exploded with orgasmic delight and my sexual energy was freed to move through my body. Darting from head to toe, womb to breasts creating ecstatic explosions like shooting stars lighting up the sky. Every cell of my being smiled with delight. My inner beauty, once muted, rose to the surface of my skin, and my face glowed radiantly. Trapped for so long, it continued to release until I felt happiness shinning from the depths of my being. My sexual energy had electrified me into an ecstatic awareness. I had never experienced anything like this before, and it felt so good.

The fierce, nourishing energy of the earth beneath my feet continued to pulse through my body. Waves of energy moved into my legs and into my womb space. It ignited my sexual energy with such a force that it pushed it into my heart, bursting it open with a rush of love. Orgasmic joy rippled through my body. I reveled in this blissful sexual energy as it streamed through my breasts, arms, lips, face, and then burst out of the crown of my head into my aura. My auric field kept expanding with my sexual energy until, I felt my consciousness connect to every star in the Milky way. In that moment I felt as if the whole universe was making love to me; I felt one with all of existence. This was the love I had always longed to feel. Inside out, I felt divine. Inside out, I shined. Inside out, I was made love to by love itself.

Intense orgasmic waves of love from the universe were brought to my body and continued for hours, days, even weeks. It was magical! It was the enlightenment I had dreamed about for years. My intuition and psychic senses activated, and I could feel healing energy pouring from my hands and body, blessing me, and life itself with beautiful vibrations. That day, my mind, heart, body, and perception of life changed. The universe had made love to me! It made me feel as if I upgraded from being a woman into being a *Goddess*. A *Goddess* in the sense that divinity united with my female form, elevating me to honour and claim myself as a sacred being. The alignment of becoming sacred, opened the gateways to perceive all of life as sacred. Everything, including myself glowed with divinity. My vibration shifted and I stepped into a world where greater love existed. In the peak of this new awareness my period began, and it was 10 days earlier than expected. I understood it to be the end of an old cycle as a woman, and the beginning of a new life cycle as a *Goddess*.

I returned home to London two weeks later. My body and aura were glowing, and I was still riding the orgasmic waves of love from the universe. I felt vibrantly alive, beautiful and super in love with all of life. It was if I was gliding through reality in my own bubble of bliss. I arrived home in the evening and I felt what seemed like an angel tap me on the shoulder and whisper, "You can't go to bed without your husband making love to you." I thought, *Yes, that's right, we should - lovemaking will bless my husband with the energy the surrounds me.'*

As we made love, I felt the divine universe buzzing around me, continuing to make love to me through my husband. I looked into my husband's eyes and made a silent prayer: "I give you this light so that you can become who you are truly meant to be." As I climaxed, I sent all the light surrounding me into my husband, I had so much of it to give. It bounced into him, lit him up, then came back into me, joining our spirits together. It was a magical moment of union that filled the entire room with light. It turned out that this was the moment I became pregnant with our beautiful baby girl, whom we would later name Aurora Elektra in honor of the energy that created her.

Before Aurora was born, I planned to have a natural "orgasmic" birth. At thirty-eight weeks, however, an ultrasound revealed that the baby was breech (feet first), and at forty-one weeks my amniotic fluid levels were so low, that I was at risk of having a stillborn baby. I had no choice but to have a Caesarean, which was not the way I envisioned my baby entering the world. I cried for hours and hours, and I wept for months after she was born. I had been robbed of my natural right as a mother to give birth the way I intended, and I felt as though my womb had been sliced in two. My sacred sexual energy collapsed along with my heart, which had been so connected to the divine universe. I was devastated. I no longer felt my radiance glowing through my being, and I no longer felt electrically alive. My sensual magic had vanished. I felt ugly.

My "soul grief" continued for months, despite the support of my husband and friends, until one day I remembered the strength I had always called on in my darkest moments. Gradually, I loved my womb back to health and healed my broken mother's heart. I loved my sexual energy to become a sacred force again, and I discovered simple exercises to help guide it up my body, through my heart, and toward the heavens - until my vibrant, orgasmic, and sensual connection to the divine universe returned. It was through this two-year healing process that I discovered that sexual energy acts as a fuel to support the love within to exist more in the body, acting like scaffolding to connect one's energy field to the heavens.

My experience of my sacred sexual energy awakening to conceive my daughter, the devastation and collapse of it through her birth, and the healing of it initiated me onto the path of sensual enlightenment – this is my sacred revolution. The wisdom I have gathered both personally and professionally is what I will share with you in this book. In addition to my own healing, each of the women I have worked with has taught me something valuable about the female body. You will learn how a woman's path toward enlightenment is a path of love. That love begins in the body so you can awaken your sexual energy as a sacred force, and powers your being to connect to the vibration of love that surrounds you. You will understand that love is the human experience of heaven and that your body becomes the vessel to create heaven on earth. This sparks your journey into sensual enlightenment – a sacred revolution where your body, heart, power and sexuality learn to unite with love. This is a path of transformation. After reading this book, you will know how to:

- Appreciate your female body as a temple and a sacred vessel of creation.
- Let your inner beauty become your outer radiance.
- Discover how sensuality is a woman's spiritual path toward enlightenment.

- Feel stable in love no matter what situation you are in.
- Generate your own supply of love inside your body.
- Feel confident and empowered by your own sexual energy.
- Reach your multi-orgasmic potential.
- Navigate through relationships and experience greater love with yourself and your partners.
- Become the powerful and magical woman that you know you already are.
- Discover how love can revolutionize your entire life.

No matter how you relate to self-love or your sexual energy, I will guide you back to the magic of your female body temple. Let me take you on a journey that will change the way you relate to your body and your life forever......

1

The Journey into Sensual Enlightenment

Women are incredible creatures and the female body is exquisite in design. We come from the stars and are made from the earth. We are of this world and at the same time we belong to the universe. No rules or laws ultimately bind us, because at the core of our being is love. We belong to love; we have come from love, and love is the direction we choose to live from. Women are the keepers of the path of love and we know it can revolutionize our lives. Love is our power; it is our wisdom and keeps us sacred. We may not always have the words to describe it, but we know it, we feel it ringing through our being.

Love makes us feel beautiful and bright, wise and empowered. It makes us intuitive, sensitive and sensual all at once. We can smell it in the air, feel it through our skin and we can spot it by looking into another person's eyes or watching their actions. Love fills us with longing and desire. It helps us manifest a reality where heaven on earth can exist. Love is our origin and our destination.

The journey into love is the path of enlightenment for a woman. This is your spiritual path. It's not a journey to meet and obey "God," but a way to unlock the mysteries of the universe. The path of love is a sensual experience, an embodiment and a love affair. It is felt through every cell in the body, and it sings through the heart, breasts, belly, womb, vagina, and through every strand of hair. The path of love is a sacred path that wills you to love every piece of yourself until you claim yourself as precious. It is the path that will turn you, beautiful woman, into a divine being—a goddess.

You are the only person in this universe that can take this path. No man, no teacher, no teaching—only you can claim yourself as a sacred being. Learn to love every thought, every emotion, and action you take. Learn to love every curve, from your hips to your breasts, on your female body. Your quest is to unlock the consciousness of your exquisite female body temple, so the divine universe can flow from the heavens, through your being, to bless and awaken life. You are here to fall in love with yourself so much, that you discover the universal vibration of loving light that exists within you. This is the same divine energy that you have been seeking outside of yourself. From the spiritual to the physical, from yourself to another, from your inner world to the outer world, from the stars to the earth. You are here to both meet and create love. From head to toe, womb to heart, body to soul, every cell in your female body is designed to blossom with the sensual enlightenment of love. Your senses will ignite and your body temple will open with the ecstatic joy of living.

Sensual enlightenment is the ability for you to fall so deeply in love with yourself that the divine universe is able to make love to you. After all, the ultimate way for a woman to create love is to be made love to, and what better partner is there than the energy of love itself. This is the "oneness" and "wholeness" and "sense of completion" you deeply desire.

Every enlightenment is an awakening that will free your mind to think beyond the normal, and at the same time it will activate your body to function in a new way. Enlightenment occurs every time you have an awareness that releases you from limitations or the experience of being trapped inside your body. Reality consists of a spectrum of vibrations that condense from the lower, loveless frequencies such as hate, revenge, and anger to the higher love-generating frequencies such as bliss, joy, and ecstasy. Every time you awaken from your density, moments of enlightenment naturally follow, which can include inspiring thoughts, a decision to change your life or behavior, visions, spiritual insights, psychic perceptions, profound orgasmic experiences, vibrational changes in the cells, and much, much more. When you learn to transduce love through your body, your consciousness will awaken, and this makes enlightenment an all-body and therefore deeply sensual experience.

"Enlightenment is an all-body and deeply sensual experience."

Sensual Enlightenment is the embodiment of heaven in a woman's body—not a destination but a complete state of being. To achieve this, sensual enlightenment requires that you marry your sexual energy to the love that exists within you. Once this occurs, the relationship with your sexual energy will change. No longer will you suppress it or give it away to serve others; instead you will use it to ignite your senses, body, heart, mind, and soul. Your sexual energy is designed to be sublimated into spiritual energy, thus making it an essential ingredient to experience enlightenment in a very physical and divinely beautiful way.

"Your sexual energy is designed to sublimate into spiritual energy."

Training your sexual energy, to travel up from your genitals to ignite your heart, will help you to love yourself until you become your own soul mate. It will also be the potent fuel that awakens your being to fall in love with life, and in return all of life will fall in love with you. Synchronicities, opportunities, and miracles will take place more easily, and your ability to manifest will improve. When your sexual energy moves toward the top of your head, you help your body to defy gravity, and this promotes anti-aging. Finally, when your sexual energy shines out of your crown and connects to the heavens, you awaken your intuitive and healing abilities. This will give you the profound spiritual insights needed to navigate through life and discover your life purpose. From this position you will be empowered to shine your magnificence and bless life wherever you go.

'Honor your inner beauty until it becomes your outer radiance.'

Sensual enlightenment encourages you—and every woman—to discover and honor your inner beauty until it becomes your outer radiance. Sensual enlightenment is a rite of passage that every woman needs in order to feel awakened. It is a beautiful and magical journey of discovering the self in a divinely feminine and deeply sensual way.

The Six Principles of Sensual Enlightenment

These six principles are the pillars that escort your journey into sensual enlightenment. Below is the overview of the principles that you will explore in more depth throughout this book. I offer it so that you can easily orientate yourself on a path that may be otherwise foreign.

1. Love is your origin and destination in all situations. *(Chapters 1, 3 & 4)*
2. Love means loving every part of your body, mind, and soul. *(Chapters 2, 6, 8, 9 & 10)*
3. Sexual energy is a sacred force that awakens your body to greater experiences of love in the physical world. *(Chapters 1, 5, 6, 12 & 13)*
4. In order to evolve, you must heal your past so the lower vibrations/feelings/memories/thoughts within can return to love. *(Chapters 7, 8 & 11)*
5. You are here to master love in all your relationships. *(Chapters 9, 10, 11 & 12)*
6. You are a creator, keeper, and lover of life, with the ability to transform and heal everything in your life to a higher vibrational state. *(Chapters 3, 4, 6, 7, 8, 11, 13 & 14)*

1. *Love Is Your Origin and Destination*

The path of sensual enlightenment is a beautiful journey that begins in your heart, travels through your body, moves through the earth, and ends in the heavens. It is a total-body experience that ignites every emotion and thought you have. As a woman, you are intricately connected to love; it lives inside every cell and fiber in your body. Your female design has evolved over millions of years to create, form, and give life. Your breasts, your womb, your vagina are all sacred portals to sustain life. You are energetically, physically, and intuitively connected to all that exists. Whether you are consciously aware of it or not, you have a very deep relationship to the fabric of life. You have the ability to create something from the nothingness. You have the ability to weave love back into the fabric of life. You have the ability, through intention, to birth the divine universe into existence. You, beautiful woman, are a gateway between heaven and earth. Your body temple is the interface between love and life.

'*Your female body is designed to birth love into life.*'

You are a walking, talking, breathing and vibrating being of love. You are of this world, and yet at the same time you belong to the divine universe. No rules or laws ultimately bind you, because at the core of your being is love. Love is your sacred source of everlasting enlightenment. You belong to love. You have come from love, and love is the direction that you choose again and again.

Love is the human experience of heaven. You are on this earth to raise the vibrations of life around you until all of life learns to resonate with love. To dance, to sing, to cry, to love, to lead, and to teach are all expressions of love that can only occur from the perspective of a physical body. Your female body is designed to birth love into life. You have an inexhaustible ability to generate love, no matter how many times you have been put down, challenged, or betrayed. The love at the core of your being lights you up from the inside and wills you—sometimes even dares you—to stand stronger, be bolder, and act kinder.

No longer will you live from a place of lack or from your insecurities. Fear, loneliness, and disappointments will always be a part of the human experience, but through the prism of love, you will recognize that every experience is designed to make you mature, grow, and blossom into more authenticity. Through love, every adversity can be used to advance you into a more profound and sublime experience of life. The more you accept the nature of your true being, the more your heart will relax and expand into the truth that the abundant reality within and beyond you is love.

You belong to the great field of love that exists infinitely everywhere. Your essence comes from this exquisite force, often called "the light." When you chose to incarnate into your body, you imprinted every cell in your being with love. Coded inside of you is all the information you require to awaken into the great field of love that surrounds you. Every spark of love that exists inside of you, is designed to connect, with every spark of love that surrounds you. Every awakening into love is an enlightenment. Every time love is felt, experienced, and generated is a moment of enlightenment.

Love is your dearest teacher, your wisest friend, and your most cosmic lover. The journey into sensual enlightenment means that you have the potential of being made love to by love itself. To fall in love with love is the most exquisite adventure you will ever have. In time, as you awaken, it will be the only experience you ever desire.

2. Love Means Loving Every Part of Your Body, Mind, and Soul

As your female body evolves and becomes a conduit of love, you will be able to pass waves and waves of love through your vessel and out into life. These waves of love are sublimely benevolent and ecstatically orgasmic, and they will make you feel so beautiful that you will glow. In order for this to occur, you must learn to love all your inadequacies and imperfections until you learn to fall in love with yourself. This is self-love, and it will ensure that you become your own best friend and your own soul mate first. Self-love teaches you how to be kind to yourself, and then you will be more compassionate with others. It releases judgments, egoic needs, and demands that would otherwise jeopardize love. When you love yourself, those around you will love themselves, and the generation of love continues and overflows.

Through the process of self-love, your body will naturally learn to generate more love. Your cells will fill with love; shining through your body from head to toe. Your inner beauty will then be encouraged to become your outer radiance. The more love you generate within, the more you will be able to expand into the love that surrounds you. Love is infinite and so are you, which makes your journey into self-love never ending. You, beautiful woman, help love to exist in the world, it begins with yourself, extends to others and through this you imprint reality to behave in brighter ways.

3. Sexual Energy As A Sacred Force

As love shines through your body, your sexual energy will start to awaken as a sacred force, that is magnetized to the love in your cells. Just like two lovers that desire to unite, your sexual energy longs to be connected to love. Since you have billions of cells that are coded with love, there are a billion places within your body that your sexual energy can magnetize. On the path of sensual enlightenment, you will learn that your sexual energy can make love to every part of your body. The love that exists in your heart, feet, legs, hands, ears, eyes, and nose can all be nourished by your sexual energy until your body blossoms with joy. Your senses will heighten, flowers will smell more magnificent, food will taste more luxurious, music will sound more alive, and spontaneous moments of joy will occur more often. From this position you will be able to entice, seduce, and encourage all of life to fall in love with you, just like you would with a lover. These are all moments of love choosing to make love to you through the experiences of everyday life. It is your sexual energy that helps love to materialize into the physical experience. It will bring to your body renewal, rejuvenation, and aliveness. Through this process, your skin will glow, your beauty will shine, and you will feel more present and empowered in your beautiful female body temple – youthful and limitless, clear and positive.

Sexual energy begins as a raw force that is driven by the instinct to procreate, but as it learns to travel up the body to meet love, it sublimates into a more refined energy. Training your sexual energy to travel up from your genitals to your heart centre, will heighten your ability to generate self-love. When your sexual energy supports your heart, you will feel more stable, less anxious, and more empowered to be more yourself. Just as a soul mate comes into your life to support, care, and strengthen you, your sexual energy does the same job. A woman who has cultivated her sexual energy into her heart, will always feel stable in the vibration of love and therefore powerful in her life. This is her own divine inner marriage. No longer will you expect others to supply you with love, because you are able to generate and ignite yourself with your own source. You won't *need* love because you already *have* it, and this will make your relationships healthier and less co-dependent.

'Your sexual energy is magnetized to love.'

Your sexual energy also becomes the potent fuel to open your heart to fall in love with life. Love shines from your cells, and your sexual energy directs it out into life. Your sexual energy provides the fuel to expand your energy field until it unites with the great field of love that surrounds you. Your sexual energy helps love blossom through your body, out to awaken life, and then up toward the heavens to accelerate your ascension. Sexual energy is therefore, the scaffolding that supports your energy body to become as big as it infinitely desires.

As your sexual energy shines from your cells into your aura, and then to the energy fields that extend beyond your body, energetic antennas form to help you intuit the environment. These antennas can extend into other dimensions and realms, and your consciousness can travel along them to pick up psychic information from other worlds and times. Since your sexual energy sublimates into spiritual energy, these antennas also sublimate into finer networks that pick up the high vibrational field of love that you came from.

From this reunion, you are able to transduce love back to your body through your sensual antennas. This can be a very orgasmic experience and can give you the sensation of being made love to by the divine universe. Through this, you will be able to harness the great field of love to arrive in your body temple. You are a gateway to bridge heaven and earth, and through this process you awaken life to operate from love. This ability means that you are active in the spiritual evolution of our planet. To be able to raise the consciousness of humanity, from the love that pours through your body temple, is an act of sensual enlightenment. Beautiful woman, love cannot exist unless you choose to embody it, and your sexual energy is the physical fuel to make this happen.

4. In Order to Evolve You Must Heal Your Past So the Lower Vibrations Within Can Return to Love

The side effect of cultivating your sexual energy is that it will begin to hit against the lower vibrations that are caught in your body. This includes old memories or traumas that are imprinted in your cells, or emotions such as guilt, shame, unworthiness, jealousy, anger, loneliness, grief, confusion, and worry. These lower vibrations have been formed from childhood experiences, relationship breakdowns, genetic traits passed down through generations, the influence of the collective consciousness, the media, and so on. The lower vibrations within you are dense and clog the energy pathways that your sexual energy must travel through. Just like a lotus that transcends from the mud to become a beautiful flower. You too, must allow your sexual energy to pass through the mud of your lower emotions and vibrational density. Your body will then be able to blossom into the experience of love.

'The lotus transcends from her mud.'

This is a beautiful process. Through the ability to evolve from your limitations, you begin to know yourself and therefore, know your purpose in every situation. When you choose to love your inadequacies, you learn to self-heal. Self-healing always leads to self-discovery, and as you discover your unique gifts and special talents, you will understand your life's purpose. Through this process, fundamental questions such as "Who am I?" and "Why am I here?" are answered, and you are able to relax in the clarity of your authentic truth, which ultimately is love.

It is your sexual energy that pulls the vibration of love through your body into the physical world. It therefore gives the love inside of you a sense of identity, and it keeps you anchored in the present so you can learn to fully exist in your body temple. Sexual energy allows you to be an individual in oneness, and this makes you a unique fractal of love. Never before and never again will the unique expression of love that emits through you exist again. The mud your sexual energy travels through to birth your version of love, and the kindness you give yourself to transcend it, creates a very special wisdom. The adversities you experience and the choices you make to overcome them imprint love with new awareness. Your unique life journey helps make the great field of love more intelligent, and this helps others to use a more brilliant love for their own evolution You, beautiful woman, heighten love because you have chosen to heal, and this is medicine for others.

5. *Master Love in All Your Relationships*

One of the sweetest adventures you will have as a woman is sharing your love with another person. Love is the human experience of heaven. It therefore requires that you learn to exchange love with other humans. The people who you choose to experience love with are your soul mates. A soul mate could be a lover, partner, friend, family member, colleague, and even a pet. Every relationship will teach you something very valuable about the mechanics and dynamics of love. The act of love involves giving and receiving words, sharing ideas, and displaying affection through touch and acts of kindness. On the path of sensual enlightenment, you will learn to master love within yourself, so you can master love with others.

To master love means that you heal all your corrupted definitions of love. Some of these might include:

"Love is painful."

"Love is abusive."

"Love always leaves."

"Love always creates fights."

No longer can you project the damaged relationship you had with your mother, father, or anyone else onto the next person. Nor can you expect another person to heal the distortions within you. As an evolved being, you must learn to self-heal, and through this process you learn to love your wounds and therefore love yourself more. When self-healing occurs, the love you have for yourself teaches you how to have compassion for others, and this will show them how to relate in a whole new way. When two people love themselves, both parties radiate love into each other; this is true love. The ability to raise your partner in love can only occur when you become your own soul mate first.

In intimate relationships your sexual energy will seek out the vibration of love that exists in your partner's body. Likewise, you will allow your partner's sexual energy to seek out the love that exists within your body. It is through this exchange that both parties activate more love to overflow into the other. When love is highly vibrating through the body, touch becomes electrifying, kisses more delicious, and sexual intimacy a beautiful interlacing of two people becoming one. Both bodies then become a superhighway for the exchange of soul information, allowing both parties to encode each other with new awareness. On the path of sensual enlightenment, you will attract people to you that have qualities you are missing and vice versa. It is through your ability to communicate and act with love, that the qualities of love will be transferred in a way where both parties can evolve. To be able to master love with another person is a pinnacle moment on the sensual enlightenment path, for love is magnified when it is duplicated (and in some cases triplicated). Love replicates infinitely, if you continuously choose to pass it on.

'Love replicates infinitely, if you continuously choose to pass it on.'

When two individuals love themselves and are able to complete themselves, this makes a relationship super juicy. Neither one is operating out of a sense of obligation or having to fill the emotional needs of the other person. Neither one has to deny who they are or live in silent resentment when they are too afraid to speak their truth. Neither one says nasty things to the other person or manipulates them in order to gain power. When two people love themselves, the relationship is healthy and vibrant. There is joy and acceptance, freedom and care, mystery and support. Such a relationship is dynamic and empowering. It is filled with wisdom and playfulness. Both partners can be fluid and open to the changing needs of the other. There is a genuine desire to support the other person to become who they truly are. When two people overflow with love for each other, a very magical relationship is created. On the path of sensual enlightenment, you will recognize that you have the ability to raise all relationships, not just those with your lover, to this heightened state of human love exchange. To live in a world where everyone you encounter is able to explore love, is the only way to truly master love. Our soul mates highlight our inadequacies, and they also show us what is missing in our lives—without them the path to enlightenment would be lonely.

6. *You Are a Creator, Keeper, and Lover of Life, with the Power to Transform and Heal Everything*

On the path of sensual enlightenment, you will learn to love everything until it becomes alive with consciousness. When this occurs, everything that surrounds you becomes an opportunity for the great field of love to communicate. Birds will sing for you, messages will be given through your surroundings, songs with meaningful words will be played, and chance meetings will be arranged for you.

'Your version of love is what this universe wants the most.'

This path will also teach you how to master your life through the virtues of love. Patience, tolerance, wisdom, courage, power, faith, forgiveness, and compassion will become your tools for communication and action. Every situation that presents itself to you will be a beautiful game. It will challenge you to apply your knowing of love, so ascension can take place. Every time you do this, you will become stronger, more stable, more centered, more beautiful, more magical and more powerful. When love becomes the core of your power, you will become more magnetic and life will realign to support and serve you. As you cherish life, life will treasure you. Creative ideas will flood your mind, inspire your heart, and your body will create your version of love in order to receive abundance. Perhaps it is writing a book, coaching someone to master their life, having a child, setting up a charity, or changing the culture in the corporation you work in. Love can be manifested in so many ways, but it is your version of love that this universe wants the most. You, beautiful woman, are required for greater love to exist.

Throughout this book you will be guided to understand and experience the six principles of sensual enlightenment. Chapter by chapter, layer by layer, petal by petal, until you blossom into the beauty that you truly are. This book is an awakening for your entire female body, heart, mind, and soul. You are invited to let the words ignite, inspire and move you. Each chapter has reflection questions that help you to grow, and movement exercises that are designed to embody the teachings. For extra support you can also access guided resources by visiting: www.vanyasilverten.com/sensual. My aim is that by the time you have finished reading this book you feel completely loved. And so we take our first step into love by celebrating your exquisite female body temple.

2

Incarnating into the Female Body

You live in a sensational female body that has the potential to flower with the cosmic and orgasmic energy of love. Every part of you—your breasts, your hair, your eyes, your hands, your feet, your womb, your vagina—are super magical. Highly intuitive and deeply sensual, your female body is exquisite in design and longs to be unlocked. The sensual magic of your body is unlocked every time you choose to awaken it with the divine consciousness that exists inside of you. Each awakening frees your mind to think beyond the normal and at the same time activates your body to function in a new way. This is how one incarnates one's soul into one's body, and this is how one embodies love as a physical experience.

Your female body temple is perfectly configured to flow with the expression of love. As a result, your love can be sultry, seductive, passionate, kind, mothering, compassionate, tender, inviting, wise, and empowering. You are powerful beyond measure, and as a woman you can never be defined or contained; you are ever changing, and ever evolving. On your quest toward your own unique enlightenment, you will dance through many emotions, many characters, and many qualities, for you are everything and anything at will, and life requires all of you to exist. Playful, wild, innocent, assertive—the list of who you are goes on forever. Let the words in this chapter awaken your body until you feel the magical qualities of your loving female power activating in all your cells.

Your Exquisite Female Body Temple

Your beautiful female body is designed to flow with the expression of love. Every step you take, every flick of your hair, and every smile you give emits love into reality. You ooze love through every pore, and like honey, your being becomes a nectar to nourish life. It is through self-love that you will learn to talk to your body like a sister, honor it like a friend, nurture it like a mother, and enjoy it like a lover. The curve of your hips, the bow in your lips, the roundness of your breasts, the bend in your back, the ovals of your eyes, the round shape of your earlobes, the swirls in your hair, the curls of your eyelashes, and the scoop in your nose[1] all portray that you have a beauty and power that is beyond measure. Your curves can both magnetize attention and act as empowered boundaries. Every one of your curves is truly exquisite—notice them all, love them, be empowered by them. They are integral to your female form.

'Your beautiful body is your guide and guru.'

Your beautiful body is your guide and guru. Any stiffness, pain, or aches is your body telling you that your consciousness is out of alignment with love. Something in your life needs to be adjusted, corrected, or examined. You will learn to welcome any ailments with joy because each one will teach you something very valuable about you and your life. Loving yourself healthy is normal when you come from love.

The more you love yourself, the more you will stimulate the love that exists in every cell to shine out and fill your body. As this occurs, all your energy pathways will begin to fill with love, and this will warm you with a sense of contentment from head to toe. As love overflows through

---

[1] Beautifully described by Mary Lofgran

your different body parts, you will notice aspects of your divine female consciousness awaken. The more love you are able to let exist in your body, the more conscious you will become.

As your breasts fill with love, you will notice an innate desire to nurture and care for life. When love shine out of your nipples, you will start to feel proud that you have the resources to make the life around you grow. When this occurs, you may notice your chest expanding, and your posture straightening in the acknowledgment that you are aligning to your truth. This will help love to burst through your throat, voice, and mouth and you will be moved to choose words that help to direct and awaken others into love. As love blooms through your ears, you will be able to hear higher vibrational guidance. When it blossoms through your eyes, you will be able to see the truth from the perspective of love. When love fuels your thoughts, it clears your mind from negative thinking, and as it extends through your hair, you will begin to feel wiser. Every hair on your head will activate, becoming little antennas so you can intuit the beautiful cosmic forces that surround you. As love runs down your spine and strengthens your bones, you will begin to feel stable and secure. As it warms your heart, your blood, and your muscles, you will notice yourself becoming more courageous. As love fills your stomach and your solar plexus, you will begin to feel both empowered and powerful. When it blossoms through your hips, you will feel like dancing, and as love wakes up your legs and feet, you will move forward knowing that more abundance can be experienced in life. As love bursts from your toes and anchors your feet to the ground, you will feel deeply connected to this extraordinary planet we live on. As love blossoms through your womb and ignites your ovaries, vagina, and clitoris, you will begin to feel empowered as a sacred sexual being who has the ability to magnificently create anything your heart desires. When your sexual energy is ignited with love, it will begin its journey of traveling and ascending up your body. This beautiful moment will ensure that your entire body is nourished by your sexual energy, and you will be able to make love to yourself.

'Your sexual energy shines love through your body.'

As your sexual energy pushes the love within to shine out from your body, you will discover what it feels like to be in love with life. A deep appreciation and immense gratitude for your existence—and all of existence—will awaken within you, and this will allow more love to flow from your being. When you allow the love within you to be fueled by your sexual energy, the more present, grounded, and centered in your body you will feel. As your sexual energy shines love out of your body, the more presence you will have to magnetize experiences of love to you physically. You birth love into your body to discover your beauty and your truth, and you birth love into life so the world can live more beautifully and more truthfully.

As your sexual energy transcends to unite with your senses and your brain, the love within your head will awaken - your thoughts will become clearer and your intuition sharper. This allows you to perceive life as a landscape of love with more ease. Love will become your core vibration, and in turn it will be reflected in physical reality. Your exquisite female body is a vessel, a conduit, and a transmitter of love. Your sexual energy will enable you to experience love as physical pleasure through your senses.

Senses and Sensuality

The greatest way to experiencing enlightenment as a sensual experience is through your five senses. Sight, smell, taste, touch, and hearing act as gateways into the physical world. These are the information gatherers of the outside world. Our senses orient us to the environment and help us make sense of life. The key to becoming more alive in your body is to live more through your senses. Being aware of your senses allows you to be more present in the now. The senses "turn the body on." Such a state heightens your experience of life, and you become more receptive to love; colors become more vibrant, sounds more beautiful, smells more fragrant, tastes more delicious— and you feel more succulent. Living in your senses amplifies life. Your senses signal aliveness and become the bridge for you to experience life—and most importantly, pleasure. You, beautiful woman, are a very sensual being, and your senses open the doors to experiencing pleasure.

As you welcome more moments of pleasure, you will learn to have a beautiful love affair with life. Pleasure requires you to slow down, be present with the environment, quiet your mind, and become more conscious of your five senses. Pleasure asks that you open your heart and put your body first as often as you can. It requires you to creatively seek and interact with life in a new way. Pleasure keeps you centered and nourished and opens the door to a new world, a world where you get to live in celebration.

With practice you will learn to cultivate the love within so it unites with your sexual energy, allowing you to ride waves of pleasure throughout the day. Every sensation of pleasure creates health, energy, inspiration, creativity, and beauty. This is the way your body temple physically manifests love. It might be a bubble of bliss that bursts through your heart, a ripple of happiness over your skin, an ecstatic joy that urges you to sing, or a sense of expanding freedom that makes you feel liberated from the density of life. It could be laughter, a gentle touch, a sensual kiss, a beautiful sound, or a delicate scent. Pleasure is registered in your physical body and grounds you so you can experience heaven on earth. When you feel pleasure in your body, it is easier to love and romance yourself. Pleasure can be found in reading a good book, enjoying drops of water splashing against your face, cuddling soft pillows, eating juicy ripe fruit, or looking at a beautiful picture.

Conscious pleasure allows you to anchor more deeply into the experience of your body in the physical world. The senses are necessary for us to experience abundance in the material world. They act as gateways to bring awareness to our bodies and new sensations to the soul. We often forget to notice our senses picking up pleasurable experiences, and thus we miss the opportunity to experience abundance in everyday life. Without your senses, you would never enjoy the wind in your hair, feel pleasure in receiving a massage, notice a diamond sparkling, smell exquisite perfume, or taste the bubbles in champagne. Your senses allow you to experience luxury, and every woman loves to be indulged. As your senses become more refined, you will be able to feel the abundance in abundance. Every day allow yourself to find new ways to indulge your senses and experience pleasure. For example, roll around naked on your sheets, cover your body in honey before taking a shower, or jump in a mud puddle with the earth squishing through your toes like liquid velvet. When you accept that you live in an infinite reality, every experience becomes new. There are a billion, million, trillion ways to experience pleasure, even if you are doing something you've done before, such as eating chocolate or brushing your teeth. The more you open your senses, the more you experience life, and this will open the door for you to have many new experiences. Love, after all, is infinite, and so too is the universe of pleasure you live in.

'The senses are necessary to experience love and abundance in the physical world.'

Sensual enlightenment depends upon your ability to tune into the frequencies of love that exist within and around you. It is only through the physical body that love becomes an embodiment. Your five senses will help you to experience love in present time reality, and this will allow it to exist more in life. As your senses refine, you will be able to experience the spectrum of love that is generated from the physical to the spiritual worlds. The five senses allow the sixth sense—intuition—to awaken. Intuition is awareness and wisdom that combines to form guidance. Your senses also work together in different ways: you can hear until you see, smell until you taste, see until you feel, feel until you know, or know until you see.

Through this process your senses will also learn to discern what love is and what love is not. Unfortunately, we still live in a world filled with hatred, crime, corruption, and illusion. As you evolve into love, the five senses will turn into your psychic system, helping you gather the spiritual information necessary to guide you away from life's distortion and to life's beauty. This might be through insights or solutions that come to you like a flash of lightning, or it might be a profound wisdom or deep knowing about how to approach a situation.

'Your body is a beautifully refined instrument.'

You, beautiful woman, are a highly intuitive and deeply sensual being! These two qualities are ultimately the same thing. When you choose to love yourself and allow the divine universe to love you, your body will blossom and become a beautifully refined instrument—an instrument that can both intuit and generate love. Every sensory perception and psychic experience will learn to coalesce in your heart, so profound awareness can be experienced. The information your senses have gathered, will then stimulate the depths of your heart to express love in wiser ways. In other words, the data your senses have gathered from the outside world will be purified by the love in your heart so that you can perceive anything that is out of alignment. It is through your heart's filter of compassion that you also receive awareness to raise the experience, obstacle, or challenge into greater love. Your senses are key in helping your entire body system to birth the consciousness of love into reality. From there your thoughts, emotions, and actions will be fueled by love, thus helping to both imprint reality and connect it back to love. This is how you become a sensual conduit of love.

Your Heart Is the Most Magical Part of Your Female Body

Your heart is the most magical part of your female body because it is the ultimate creator and generator of love. As you awaken, you will notice yourself operating more and more from the wisdom of your heart. Your choices, thoughts, intuitions, and actions will all come from your heart and be powered by love. The greatest lesson you will learn is to have compassion and tenderness for everything, especially yourself. This is not an easy task, as life can present many so-called obstacles that trigger the limitations within, keeping your heart and cells closed to the experience of love. Every obstacle, situation, person, and experience is an opportunity to learn a lesson of love. Through every lesson of love, you will find that there is no such thing as "black or white," "good or bad," "right way or wrong way," or "guilt or drama." The mind drops its judgment and frees your consciousness, to move from your head into your heart, where the state of permanent awareness resides.

When you live from your heart, you can find blessings in hurt, relief in confrontation, joy in sadness, and opportunities in any suffering. Living from your heart allows you to live in gratitude and wonder. Idle moments are never wasted, because the joy in your heart beckons you to live more. You are able to notice the magic of life happening within and around you. You begin to see miracles in every moment. You become aware that the universe is supporting you. You learn that life is always willing you to succeed and grow. The journey into your heart is the only true pilgrimage.

'The journey into your heart is the only true pilgrimage.'

Your female heart has an enormous capacity to feel, know, sense, and understand. It is innately intuitive, compassionate, and inexhaustible.

It has an extraordinary capacity to love. Your path into sensual enlightenment will teach you how to love yourself and beyond. Your heart will give relentlessly and has an enormous desire to create harmony. The insatiable longing of your female heart desires to embrace everything until all is loved and there is peace.

But if your heart has been betrayed, you many become wild and filled with revenge. When love breaks, you break, you die inside, and may be left feeling rejected and unworthy. Over time, as the innocence of your heart breaks, you learn that love is not an external force but an internal one. Every time your heart breaks, the pain of loneliness will force you to love yourself back to health. It teaches us that we can heal and that nobody in this world can love us as truly as ourselves.

'Love is a woman's superpower.'

The heart of a woman is the most beautiful part of her being, and there is nothing more appealing than being in the presence of a loving person. Your feminine heart seeks to be deeply nourished, and self-love will become the only path to ensure it. Love is a woman's superpower. It is *your* superpower.

Self-Love Is Your Superpower

The most potent force you have available is self-love. To love yourself is to know love in the most profound way. The divine birthed itself into creation through love, and it is self-love that will birth your soul. On the path into sensual enlightenment, you will love yourself into existence. Every part of you that is hidden, denied, lost, confused, numb, or afraid will be nurtured until it shines. Self-love is not a one-time event; it is something you choose again and again. Through the process of loving your shadows, you will learn much about yourself and the nature of love. To deeply accept who you are is the most liberating, most freeing, most pleasurable experience and evolution you can have.

Self-love is the greatest gift you can give yourself. It is the sweetest, richest, deepest, most luscious, most luminous, most luxurious, most vibrant gift of them all. Loving yourself will make you a pure vessel so your higher self and the divine universe can connect and live through you. Self-love will improve your life by shifting the way you relate to your body, health, money, manifestations, creativity, and relationships. It will change your inner landscape—and therefore change the way you relate to reality.

It is only through loving yourself that you will learn to live in alignment with your true nature. Self-love means loving the entirety of who you are. Perceiving some parts of you as acceptable and repressing other parts is toxic to your system. Self-love will teach you how to live authentically and remember the simplicity of what feels good and what does not. This will evolve into your big "yes" and your big "no" as to why you do and do not do certain things. Self-love will move you into wholeness because it will teach you how to embrace and love all of your experiences and emotions, no matter how dark and troubling they have been. You'll discover that self-acceptance is the cure for shame, comparison, and jealousy. Self-love will teach you how to love your wrinkles, your cellulite, and even the mean, ugly, angry and crazy parts of you.

Self-love will ensure that you remain empowered and authentic in your relationships. You will preserve your dignity and integrity in every situation, and this will ensure that you remain aligned to the values of love. Self-love will be the safeguard that helps you navigate through all the trials and tribulations life presents you. It will inspire you to change and recreate life until it truly honors you. Self-love will make you beautiful from the inside out. It will give you a glow that radiates your unique presence into this world. As you learn to generate your own love from within - in this ever changing world, self-love will be the most guaranteed love in human form. Relationships will come and go, but self-love will always remain.

'Self-love opens the door for more love to flow to you.'

Self-love is the key that unlocks the endless fountain of love that surrounds you. Through it you will discover that you are powerful and sensual, wise and beautiful, courageous and magical. As you love yourself, you are actually allowing the great field of love that surrounds you to love you as well. Self-love opens the door for more love to flow to you. The process of self-love empowers every cell in your body to receive universal love, just as a flower drinks in sunlight to grow. The sensual expression of your body depends upon the omnipotent force of love to literally make love to your body so that it can awaken. The combination of being able to love yourself, plus being open to the vibration of love loving you, activates the magical and orgasmic qualities of your female body.

An orgasm is simply waves of ecstasy that ripple through the body. From an enlightened position, it depends on no one, because every orgasmic experience encourages the body to open like a flower, allowing your spirit to ripple through you in the delight of being alive. This is the vibrancy we all seek. The more present you are with the experience of love, the more vital and energetic you will feel as a woman.

Through this book you are invited to fall in love with yourself so much, that waves of joy flow from you to awaken the world around you. No longer do you have to wait until retire, or have a day off, or go on a vacation, or when the house is clean, or the kids are in bed. This journey begins as soon as you choose to love your exquisite female body temple. Over the next four chapters, you will learn how the vibration of love and your sacred sexual energy, unite to make this happen.

Reflection:

1. Close your eyes and feel your body. What parts naturally feel the most beautiful? What parts feel the most powerful?
2. Which parts feel shy, ugly, hidden, or rejected?
3. What would happen if you loved those parts of you? How would you feel?
4. Reflect upon the ways that self-love is your greatest superpower.
5. What would happen if you chose to love yourself more than anyone else can?
6. Your senses are the gateway to experiencing more pleasure. List twenty activities that bring you sensory pleasure on a daily basis.
7. What would happen if your body could spontaneously blossom with the ecstatic, joyful, and orgasmic experience of love?
8. What would your life be like if you allowed every moment to be a sacred blessing?

3

What Is Love?

*L*ove is defined in the dictionary as "a strong feeling of affection or attraction." This may be true as a response, but love as a state of being is far more exquisite and sublime in nature. It is a zestful, playful, and profoundly wise energy that is both fiercely courageous and touchingly tender. Many before you have followed the trail of love and discovered it as a way to master an otherwise chaotic experience of humanity. These people felt love as a sense of purity that expanded within them; it energized their body with beauty and ignited their minds with wisdom. It gave them a glowing presence that radiated through their words and actions, and it blessed those around them so they could recognize love as well. These people learned to honor love as a path toward enlightenment; they have been called saints, sages, earth angels, and light workers—you may even recognize yourself as one. Enlightenment is a spiritual journey of insight and awareness that transforms one's consciousness from suffering to peace. Love is the bridge to enlightenment, and at the same time it *is* the enlightenment. Love is the masterful key that can be applied to any situation to obtain harmony. Love knows no boundaries, holds no judgments or prejudices, is unable to reject or exclude. It cannot be bought, hidden, or denied. Love is the glue that unites all living things, and so you are never separate to all that is but rather an integral part of it. Love is available to every single person at every moment.'

As a woman, you have deep desire to become the shining brilliance of love. Now, in this quest you may experience love in confused and distorted ways or seek "love" in activities that destroy the values love upholds. But nonetheless, the desire to obtain love coupled with the pain of not fully obtaining it will force the lower parts of the self to evolve so you can meet love. For some this can be a very painful but necessary journey, but each of us must learn that beyond our limited perception is a reality far more exquisite than we could ever dream up. Confronting your limitations is what love does best. It will make you become aware of your selfish nature, your jealousy, your anger, your bitter and twisted needs, your vanity, your greed and laziness—but this is all part of love's plan to help you awaken. Your ego creates the challenge, love provides the path, and the journey toward enlightenment begins.

There are many events that break the heart, and I often reflect on my childhood years as the time when this occurred the most for me. My parents first split up when I was five years old, and then permanently when I was eight. Both parents remarried and then divorced, and as a result I had to form relationships with step-parents and step-siblings only for those to break up. This cycle continued, as my mother had four marriages and my father three. By the time I left university, I had lived in eight different family scenarios. Each time a family unit was formed, my heart made connections to form a relationship. Then when it fell apart, I had to deal with the grief and confusion of losing love. My family turmoil created much chaos. We moved often, and I went to ten different schools, changing fourteen times because I would move back and forth between families. Each time this happened, I had to make friends only to lose them again and again. I experienced heartbreak on top of heartbreak, so much so that my heart closed and became so numb that I was unable to cry for years.

'Love is available to every single person at every moment.'

I witnessed the many ways love could form between people, and I also witnessed the many ways people could destroy love through their words and actions. My childhood story gave me an intensive crash course into the fragility of the human heart and the damage it created in relationships and people's life choices. The love dysfunction I experienced taught me how to be kind, how to be independent, how to be courageous, and how to not to create hurt in others. My childhood broke me until I learned to rely on the love that existed within me first, so that I could find the real love that existed beyond me.

My heartbreaks taught me to understand when someone lied, manipulated, or tried to control me. Being heartbroken taught me that I could generate my own love and my own connection to the love that exists around me, which could never be broken. Ten years after leaving school, I became a professional intuitive healer, and I discovered that 90 percent of my client's problems stemmed from a broken heart. My experience of having my heart broken in many different ways made me understand each client's heartbreak story better. As I learned to guide myself out of my experiences, I could also guide my clients back to health.

This life will generate an infinite amount of opportunities, challenges, and experiences so you can meet and master love in all its forms. Love is a nectar that is so pleasurable and so gratifying that it will spur you on until you find and experience it. It will challenge you and at times may make you go crazy with the thought of losing it. Love will make you cry; it will make you laugh, it will make you soft, and it will make you tough.

Love is a verb, and it expresses itself through touch, words, actions, inner joy, vitality, and smiles. You will feel it shimmering through your skin, lighting up your eyes, dancing through your hips, and rippling through your lips. Love becomes a form of discipline, and you will use it to set boundaries when necessary. There will be times when you give love relentlessly, while at other times you will have to set limits around the love given in order to help someone else grow. Through your life experiences, you will learn that love is the ultimate lesson in every situation and sometimes the journey can be painful and challenging. But the more love is understood and mastered, the more authentic and more beautiful you become.

'Love is a creative force that gives birth to many virtues.'

Love is unconventional. It can never be ordered; it is a creative force that gives birth to many virtues; it is a wisdom not bound by rules.

Love only knows one thing: to meet and unite with more love. Love is a motion, and its only quest is to blossom from individuality to oneness. With this understanding, you will become aware that each virtue love generates is a brilliant facet offering a gateway to make sense of love as a totality. Every time you embrace and embody a quality of love, you naturally transcend. Transcendence is the ability to evolve out of limited thinking, distorted emotions, and destructive desires. Through this process there is a shift from life being experienced as "hell" to being lived as "heaven." The dualistic concept of hell versus heaven, light versus dark, does not actually exist when you recognize love as the bridge that unites all polarities. In fact, it is the ability to bridge all the polarities and contradiction within that stabilizes you as an individual in oneness.

When you love, your authentic self can express itself. You are no longer searching; instead, you are discovering a life that mirrors your truth. In other words, you know who you are and why you are here. The great mystery is finally solved - love leads you to your authentic self, then shows you how to act in a world so more love can flow into existence. This continuous cycle of meeting, uniting and birthing love is what a woman does best.

Through this cycle you contribute to the universal field of love that surrounds all of life. Your participation in love helps to generate more love into existence. Not only do you help to create it, but your body becomes the interface that helps to birth the heavenly dimension of love. The great field of love surrounding you is your mother, father, lover, friend, and guide—it is your cosmic family, and every quality you need to transform the human experience comes from it. Although the qualities that uphold love can never be fully comprehended, the movement of love can be broken down into thirteen main virtues.

'Love is an infinite force and its dynamic nature is limitless.'

Once you master these virtues, you will almost certainly discover more. Love is an infinite force and its dynamic nature is limitless. Are you ready to experience the magnitude of love? As you journey through the rest of this chapter, I invite you to let the words ignite your entire being. You might feel energy dip and rise inside of your body, your mind may awaken with new thoughts, or your spirit may vibrate with a deep sense of knowing. Allow this chapter to be a recognition that connects you to the transcendental awareness that you, beautiful woman, are a conduit of love.

The Thirteen Virtues of Love

1. *Ecstasy*

Love spins in ecstatic joy and creates light within your cells and joyfully tells you that you are divine. Love is completely in love with itself, and this generates an overwhelming excitement for existing. To be bursting with love and exploding with joy teaches us three very valuable things:

1. Love is an omnipotent force that has the ability to override and over power everything else. Just like a bud being willed by the sun to blossom, likewise love also acts like a force of transformation. Limited thinking cannot be sustained when joy ripples and informs that everything is in perfection.

2. In order to maintain extreme ecstasy, love fuels itself with the vibrant desire to give and receive love. It is a self-fulfilling movement that acts as a continuous rebirth into love. This somersault into and from love teaches us that love is both a celebration and a point of origin.

3. The source of self is love. Love is our parent and love is our child. Love is both the rebirth and the transcendence which gives rise to being blissfully in love. The eternal goal that every spiritual being seeks to master. To experience the ecstatic expression of love, is to arrive home. This is your spiritual destiny.

2. *Wonder*

The ecstatic experience of being in love, shifts into wonder, once there is a recognition beyond being blissfully fulfilled by love more life exists. Wonder first begins with reverence and a deep appreciate for the magnitude of love, and in that moment, one also discovers how unfamiliar love is. There is a shift from being completed by love to the realization that beyond the self, there is infinitely more love to explore and fall in love with. This moment of wonder is the first time a sense of individuality develops. This is not "I am separate from love," but rather "I am surrounded by love." Such an understanding immediately places the "I" in a completely abundant universe. From this stance of abundance, one develops trust in the unknown. The enormity of such a realization brings immense gratitude, and the awareness that develops is total awe. Could there possibly be an infinitely more exquisite form of love than me? A curiosity develops, and the need to experience love beyond myself forms. The tenacity of wonder discovers freedom, and so the journey back into oneness begins.

3. *Freedom*

Unbound to anything other than the desire to move beyond the self, the freedom of love offers an expansion into life. Not constrained by rules, regulations, or judgments, the freedom of love seeks to move from the singular to the infinite. The curiosity to discover the surrounding abundance ignites an impulse, a movement of energy that transports the self into new territories. The movement of freedom is a rite of passage that requires one to leave with no expectations other than awe and arrive with nothing other than joy. This awareness is essential, for freedom operates without attachment. If one can master entering and exiting each moment in love, a liberation into a greater experience can occur. Freedom then becomes a journey of transformation; it initiates adventures so the self can experience the magnitude of love.

4. *Desire*

Freedom initiates the wondrous journey into love, and such an exploration only ignites one thing: desire! Desire is the longing for union with that which is beyond the sense of self. It is the longing to connect and return to wholeness. There is so much eagerness in this moment that desire gives love a magnetic charge. An attraction develops, ecstatic excitement is felt, and a sense of purpose is given. Connectivity becomes both the motivation and the direction the self needs. The combination of intention with the anticipation of an unknown union becomes a tantalizing moment for love. It brings the awareness of "who am I now" and "who will I be" after the exchange. Desire is a powerful moment that says yes to becoming more. Desires motivates the self into meeting its destiny.

5. Exchange

Through desire, the self arrives at its destination, which is uniting with more love. This union begins as soon as both parties exchange their individual experience of love. This exchange is founded on the ability to share, whether ideas, experiences, needs, or desires. The exchange also requires the ability to receive, and this includes listening, holding a space so the other can express themself fully. The giving and receiving continues until both parties ignite the other into a greater sense of fulfilment. It is the moment where the self recognizes that "because of you, I am greater." This naturally develops into such a deep sense of gratitude that the self can only choose to keep giving so the other can feel greater too. The exchange of love creates a friendship, where both parties harmonize into togetherness. The birth of kindness, tolerance, cooperation, and encouragement become new sources of love, and harmony between both parties is sustained. These qualities become the tools to ensure that each aspect is always birthed into a greater sense of love by the other.

6. Generosity

In the exchange of loving each other more and more, generosity naturally develops. Generosity is the act of selflessly giving to the other without the expectation of return. Love itself bursts through any sense of control and gifts the receiver. The sheer joy of giving generates more love, and the cycle of generosity continues. This movement brings an awareness that there is more ecstatic joy in giving than holding onto things. You do not fully realize yourself until you have shared yourself fully with another person. Being generous helps the self to discover itself; every time it gives, a beautiful sense of pride emerges. This pride is not arrogant, but rather embodies self-esteem; it says, "When I give, I matter." This forms an identity aligned to the core values of love. The ability to be selfless and at the same time aware of oneself is an important balance.

The two must exist simultaneously, for giving also requires the ability to receive generosity from another.

7. Compassion

When one acts from a stance of generosity, compassion naturally follows. Compassion is an outpouring of love that does not discriminate; it is unconditional and continuous. It is the ability to see another person for all that they are and still maintain ecstatic joy. Compassion does not collapse into comparison, judgment, or defensiveness. Compassion brings openness and acceptance, allowing others to be fully in their truth even if it conflicts or does not resonate with us. It offers a psychic depth that sees beyond one's own paradigm and beyond the other's paradigm. Compassion always returns one to the purity of love within every living thing. It allows us to witness all that is out of alignment with love, and at the same time, it encourages us to heal through unconditional love. It is a love that is both tender, sensitive, and irrefutably kind. Compassion matures one's awareness.

8. Wisdom

Through compassion, wisdom naturally is born. Wisdom is acquired every time one expands into love and an adjustment in perception occurs. The wisdom of love is illuminating knowledge that offers both discernment and the way to evolve into higher consciousness. Wisdom occurs when one recognizes that they are out of alignment with love and simultaneously has an awareness of the solution that will transform one's being back to love. This process can happen quickly, leaving one with an unwavering knowing of the truth. Truth is what we all search for—it is the wisdom that completes the puzzle and makes sense of everything. Truth rings through our bones and shows us the way forward. Love is truth, and love's wisdom brings the discernment required to access it. Wisdom is acquired over time, and intelligence develops every time one orders their perceptions back to love. Through this process one generates a knowledge that provides the solutions to help others evolve into love. This is the same wisdom that all the great sages and saints possess. Every person who has birthed love's wisdom gifts the collective consciousness with a new awareness. Remember that love is an ever-evolving force that is continuously becoming more intelligent every multidimensional microsecond. This means that if you become conscious of the knowledge love holds, you can transform with every breath you take.

9. Dignity

The wisdom of love crystallizes into a moral code and provides one with an internal structure of conduct. This is not a set of rules or laws that govern one's life but rather a framework to ensure the integrity of love. The dignity of love develops when one recognizes that certain values must be respected. Love is so exquisite and so precious that it absolutely deserves to be honored. The dignity of love is a personal stance, and every individual holds a unique perspective of how love should be maintained. This is because no two journeys will ever generate the same experiences. The dignity of love is therefore sustained by an infinite amount of values. This transforms love from being an ethereal to a physical experience, giving the self a definite foundation of behavior from which to act. The dignity of love brings the awareness that love can only be maintained through right action. The self quickly learns that in order to manifest love, one must operate within a certain framework of ethics. Dignity offers the self a position of stability, order, authenticity, and integrity. The dignity of love therefore ensures that one remains true to one's specific version of love.

10. Courage

The combination of dignity, wisdom, ecstatic joy, compassion, wonder, and generosity creates an exceptionally potent force that will uphold love in all situations. Filled with a sense of responsibility, love's courage is unstoppable. Courage brings boldness and a sense of confidence, and it turns love into a powerful force that fearlessly maintains the other values of love. Courage develops as soon as the self comprehends that love is a sacred force of divinity that needs to be preserved in all circumstances. Courage brings a sense of purpose that motivates the self to protect, defend, and serve the qualities of love so love can continue to expand. The courage of love turns the self into a warrior that is brave, compassionate, and tenacious. It strengthens the self's identity and dilutes the ego. Courage offers determination and resilience in adversity.

It brings the assurance that one is undoubtedly able to raise the loveless into love. Love's courage knows that everything can be brought back into alignment through action.

11. Faith

Faith and courage tend to dance together to ensure that love comes in existence. Courage motivates one to uphold love through action, and faith motivates the action even when the outcome is uncertain. Faith is an inspiriting aspect of love; it brings the insight that there is always a more enlightened stance that can be achieved. The essence of faith comes from deep within where the full knowing of love exists. As it radiates through the body, there is a desire to find that love externally. Like a compass, faith points one in the direction of love; it guides the self to love regardless of obstacles and challenges. Faith teaches us that no adversity can hinder us from meeting love. It teaches us to completely trust that all types of experiences will eventually lead to a higher understanding of love. Faith brings joy and a knowing that all will play out perfectly if one keeps surrendering to the values of love. Just as a flower opens to the sun, faith encourages us to keep expanding into the experience of love. Love's faith brings the awareness that at every moment help, guidance, inspiration, wisdom, and grace are available. We are never alone, always supported, and completely taken care of. Faith brings the ecstatic hope that love can be experienced and created everywhere.

12. Harmony

Having faith naturally tunes one into the harmony of love. Harmony is the ability for everything, including that which has chaotic origins, to reorganize and evolve into a peaceful state. The movement into harmony is the direction that love desires. This is because love always strives for unity, and the only way it can be achieved is if the self is able sustain equality with all that exists beyond itself. Such a state requires that one is in complete balance both internally and externally. No longer can one hold judgments that define the self as superior, nor can one become isolated in inferiority complexes. Instead one must learn to create an equilibrium with all of creation. This is a position of mastery, for the self is able to maintain its uniqueness and at the same time merge into oneness.

This state allows one to feel love for itself while simultaneously feeling love for everything else. It gives rise to the awareness of being in love, for nothing is able to contradict the peaceful beauty harmony offers. The harmony of love is stable and teaches us that all we can ultimately experience is complete wonder and appreciation for all of existence. Appreciation gives birth to gratitude, the ecstatic joy of being alive. Gratitude only motivates the self to bless life with more love, and this act of generosity nourishes, stabilizes, and harmonizes our existence into a deeper experience of love. The harmony of love brings the awareness of completion, satisfaction, and contentment. It reminds us that everything exists in complete perfection. This awareness acts as a gateway into enlightenment, which is the full comprehension of love as an omnipotent and omnipresent force.

13. *Creation*

For us to feel content in a universe that is exquisitely perfect, we must learn to master the ability to create more love. This ability only occurs when the self has embodied all the qualities that love generates. To create is more than merely a transference of energy; it is a combination of genius and a wondrous desire that says, "Because of my uniqueness, I can make love more profound." This doesn't come from the perspective that the self is better than love. But rather from the awareness that the self is so in love with love, that the only way it can make love more outstanding, is to "make love" with love. This movement is extremely exciting; it stimulates both parties with all the qualities of love and initiates a frenzied transference of love. Each gives and receives, receives and gives, both creating a dynamic force of energy that collides, explodes, and initiates more love to exist. These moments create little "big bangs"—love giving birth to more love.

The sparks of energy that are created in such moments are perceived as light. This light has been known as Source, God, Allah, the Divine, etc. The light is actually love making love to itself, thus creating more love. This is an orgasmic, joyful experience of enlightenment. To both master and create love graduates the self into the ultimate purpose of expanding love. As the self matures in its ability to create love, it eventually learns to give purpose to its creation. Inspired by a higher vision of love, the self learns to nurture and lead its creations to keep ascending. Through this process, the self indirectly learns to lead and nurture itself toward ascension. The creator and the creation, the teacher and the student, the lover and the loved all exist simultaneously together. Both are creating the other to be better. This produces the sweet awareness of community and the recognition that all creations must be designed to benefit the greatest good of all. The self ascends into a more profound experience of love through creation and then expands even more through the awareness of community. Creating and connecting to more and more love returns the self to the ecstasy of love. And so the cycle of love infinitely continues with awakenings into a more profound experience of love every multidimensional microsecond. Such an exquisite dance creates the dimension of heaven.

‘The exquisite dance of love creates the dimension of heaven.’

Love is a potent force that protects you as a sacred being. It is a dynamic energy that is both multifaceted and multidimensional. It is ever changing, ever learning, ever merging, and ever ascending into a more refined experience of love. As a woman, you comprehend love as a dynamic force of virtues. You are able to hold all of its qualities, and at the same you are able to command any of them to be more present at any one time. Just as a tailor chooses various colors to make a tapestry, you too are able pull the threads of love—wisdom, courage, beauty, and desire—to create a more joyous experience. As a woman, you have the ability to float within the ocean of love, and because of this you have access to an extraordinary pool of energy. This is where you get your true power and magic. The ever-occurring blossoming into a more profound experience of love is the orgasmic awakening of enlightenment that every single cell in your body yearns for. To fall in love with LOVE is the ultimate key to experience sensual enlightenment.

One of my most sensual, enlightening, and empowering moments occurred one day when I just decided that the great field of love needed to make love to me. Usually I wait until such moments occur naturally, but on this particular day I was feeling fiery and decided that I also had the right to request a sensual awakening. So I said a prayer at lunchtime, telling the universe it needed to make love to me at sunset (which is my favorite time of the day). When dusk came, I lit some candles, put on my favorite music, and surrounded my bed with crystals and rose petals. I am definitely one for ritual, because ritual creates a sacred space within which a vortex of magical energy can exist. Every ritual also acts as gateway to step out of an old world into a new one. So before I lay down on the bed, I performed a ceremony with sacred intention. As I took off my clothes, I also stripped off the thoughts, emotions, and perceptions I no longer wanted. With every item of clothing, I also removed layers of my ego. I placed those clothes and the past outside my room, and then closed the door.

I knelt down before the bed and welcomed the vibration of love to become more present in the room. I could feel love's joy dancing around and touching my skin. I smiled, and love smiled back at me. Rubbing oil between my hands until it was warm and emitted its rose fragrance, I breathed it in and then oiled my body with it. With beautiful strokes and loving caresses, I honored my being with self-love. As I touched my skin, I intended every cell in my body to open so I could receive more love. Every touch stimulated the energy pathways in my body to awaken, and I could feel love beginning to flow through me. My body was being prepared so the entire universe could make love to me. Placing my hands in prayer, I welcome more love in the room and witnessed it sparkle across the bed. As gracefully as I could, I lay down on my bed. Love danced around me and through me.

Delightful sensations began to ripple through my body. Little orgasms popped and fizzed in my cells, and I smiled in joy. The more I opened my body to receive love, the more I noticed the vibration of love intensifying around me. My toes, which are super sensitive, began to notice the waves of love being sent from heaven. Love rippled through my feet and up my legs, hips, inner thighs, and into my vagina, which was waiting to be nourished. My fingers also drank in those waves of love to fill my energy pathways all the way to my breasts. My vagina flowered with love; my breasts blossomed with joy. The rest of my cells began opening to the waves of love being sent from the universe into my body.

Beautiful energy dipping and rising within, my spine snaked, my back arched, and my fingers curled with the intensity. The more my body opened like petals opening to the sun, the more love I could receive. As the waves got stronger and bigger, my body began to ride the ripples of love that danced through my body. I felt so much joy as love from the universe entered and exploded through my cells. I laughed, sang, and sighed as the universe made love to me. Nourished from head to toe, womb to heart, body to soul, as the love inside of me peaked, I felt completed. With every inhale I returned to love, and with every exhale I melted deeper into the exquisite vibration. Inhaling and exhaling, inhaling and exhaling, I eventually lost all sense of self and rebirthed as someone new— someone that had experienced a love that required only the willingness of my body to open to that which already exists.

As the waves subsided, my body relaxed into the gentle afterglow of lovemaking. My skin sparkled, my breath tasted sweet, and my body occasionally twitched as the last orgasmic responses faded. I felt beautiful and alive, deeply satisfied, and I experienced a sense of liberation by beckoning to the divine universe to complete me. This moment of sensual enlightenment taught me that at any time, I can request to be made love to by love itself.

> **'Self-love is a gift you consciously choose
> to give yourself again and again.'**

As a woman, your body is intricately connected to the vibration of love. It glows in your cells and is coded in your DNA. You have a psychic, telepathic, and energetic connection to the divine universe. Your body is like a cosmic flower—all your energy pathways are rooted in love, and you are able to drink in these very nourishing vibrations to feed your cells. When you feel completely nurtured by love, your cells blossom and feed the rest of your body this very beautiful energy. This is an act of self-love, a gift you consciously choose to give yourself over and over again—until every thought is fueled by love, every emotion concludes in love, and every action promotes love in the physical world. Self-love fuels the energy pathways to become more active and vibrant. It awakens the higher intelligence within the DNA to exist so the ego can deflate, and it encourages your unique beauty to unfold. This blossoming is orgasmic in nature, and the sensations of joy, ecstasy, bliss, and beauty flower through your body every time you choose love.

Reflection:

1. Which virtue/quality of love excites you the most? Why?
2. Which virtue/quality of love do you feel you have mastered? Why?
3. Which virtue/quality of love feels the most foreign to you?
4. Which virtue/quality of love do you long for the most?
5. What would happen to your body if you mastered all the virtues/ qualities of love?
6. What would happen to your mind if you mastered all the virtues/qualities of love? How would it change the decisions you make? How would it help your relationships? Your ability to communicate?
7. What are the greatest memories you have on experiencing love? This could include your childhood, your relationships, or everyday life.
8. Reflect upon love itself making love to you. Explain the sensations and the experience.

4

Riding the Orgasmic Waves of Love

The dictionary defines an orgasm as the physical and emotional experience at the peak of sexual excitation, usually resulting from the stimulation of the sexual organs. But orgasms are so much more! They come in many forms, they can range from subtle to strong; they can be any release of energy from the inside to the outside of your body. And while most of us believe that the genitals have to be involved, you can also achieve an orgasm through the sheer power of your mind, senses, and the will of your heart.

Orgasms help birth the energy of love through the physical body. Since love is infinite, there are as many different types of orgasms as there are stars in the sky. You can have an orgasm when you are touched or while you are looking at flowers, smelling perfumes, or brushing your hair. Some women have orgasms when they give birth. They can occur while dancing as pleasurable sensations move through your body. You might feel a tingle in your hands or lips, a ripple of joy, euphoria, waves of peace and pleasure, or an electrical current shooting through your body. Orgasms can be compared to riding a roller coaster of bliss. Up, down, and around; sensations travel through your body as your sexual energy darts in different directions, igniting the love that exists inside of you. In high peaks of arousal, you can experience hundreds of ecstatic vibrations traveling through your body.

Like my experience in the rainforest just before I conceived my daughter, your sacred sexual energy will provide the fuel to help you connect to the vibrations of love that come from the universe, both within and around you. Remember that your sexual energy is attracted like a magnet to love. The more love you generate and connect to, the more your sexual energy will be attracted to it. This is why when a woman makes love, she opens her whole being so her partner's sexual energy can find the love that exists within her. This exchange of energy is why a woman tends to fall in love with the person she has been intimate with. Likewise, such an experience can be had with your own sexual energies uniting with the love that exists within your own body. An orgasm is simply the physical manifestation of love that uses your sexual energy to pass through your being; it can be localized to an all-body experience, including just yourself or extending to others and beyond.

The Connection Between Orgasms and Love

Because you are made up of billions of cells from head to toe, womb to heart, body to soul, your sexual energy has the potential to infuse your entire body are create the physical experience of love. Through practice, you can learn how to summon your sexual energy and feel it travel and vibrate through the cells in your body. If you like, you can view the love in your cells as being feminine in nature, and your sexual energy as being masculine. Love has the desire to nourish, and sexual energy has the desire for freedom—an exquisite combination that completes and transforms the other into higher vibrational experiences. This begins the process of sexual energy sublimating into spiritual energy, creating a state of vibrancy and rejuvenation in the body, mind, heart, and soul.

Like two lovers who want to get to know one another more intimately, your sexual energy "makes love" to your cells. In response, your cells blossom with an orgasmic expression of love. Eventually your entire body is flooded with love, and all the cells and energy pathways are filled to the point where they begin to radiate out into the universe. Imagine this: your fingers, eyes, ears, mouth, nose, breasts, nipples, hips, vagina, and toes all orgasm with love. This is when your inner beauty becomes your outer radiance, which you will discover in chapter six – *The Art Of Blossoming*. It is a joyous moment, and it feels like a release. Finally, the essence of who you truly are is freed, and the love of the universe is able to pass through you as waves of joy, pleasure, liberation, and celebration. From your body into the world, into your partner (if you have one), nourishing all life around.

Every orgasm, therefore, is a blossoming of love from your inner self to the outer world, but the greatest orgasms can happen when your sexual energy is released from your body into the field of love that surrounds you. When this occurs, your sexual energy can transduce universal love back into your body. In doing so, you call the orgasmic waves of love that emit from the divine universe to make love to every part of you. Such an experience is extremely healing, for it teaches you what it feels like to be completely loved by all of life. This is an essential moment on the path of sensual enlightenment - opening yourself to receive more love, increases your capacity to love yourself, and this makes you a bigger vessel to receive more love from the universe. And this cycle never ends; it goes on and on with profound awakenings into a greater understanding of love. Enlightenment is infinite and so too is the experience of love from the perspective of your exquisite female body.

Orgasms can be Healing, Rejuvenating, and Enlightening

Orgasms may feel sexual or they may not, but they certainly arouse your senses so you can experience the vibrancy of life. Sometimes orgasms can be painful. If this happens, it is your sexual energy moving through your repressed emotions or old hurts in your body. When the orgasm pushes through such blocks, there is an enormous relief, followed by renewal. In this way, orgasms can be simultaneously healing, rejuvenating, and enlightening. They are magical, and they can bring on visions, psychic perceptions, profound spiritual insights, vibrational changes in our cells, and even restore health to your body.

As you awaken to your orgasmic potential, you become more

receptive to the infinite amount of ways, love can pass through your body, mind, soul, and life. Every orgasm you have is an opportunity for the dynamic "virtues of love" to collide inside of you. Like a cyclical pinball machine of love, ecstasy collides with freedom, which unleashes desire, which ignites passion, which cascades into harmony, which arouses ecstasy again. It is the most pleasurable way to let go of your old identity and limitations, and it's an exciting way to understand that both the self and life are one divine experience of orgasmic love. Each orgasm is a moment of enlightenment freeing you from the illusion that you are trapped inside your body. The more your sexual energy is freed to travel through your body, the more it will be able to travel through your energy field and beyond to the heavens. This offers the oneness that you seek on your spiritual path. It's not a destination, but an embodiment of love manifesting throughout reality. It is your sexual energy that supplies the fuel to make this connection.

The Wild, Wild World of Orgasms

Since there are infinite ways love can be orgasmically experienced, let's explore the different types of orgasms you can have, from the microscopic to the cosmic.[2] As you read the descriptions below, allow your sexual energy to ignite and be open to the ecstasy you can experience from it. Feel the sensations of love as your sexual energy dips and rises, dances and explodes along with the words!

Vaginal/G Spot/Cervical/Blended Orgasms
You can experience a whole array of inter-vaginal orgasms. Each area can feel slightly different, and orgasms can occur one at a time or all together. They can range from subtle to overwhelming, and from being localized (in areas such as the cervix or clitoris) before extending through the body and activating other areas such as the nipples. Vaginal orgasms can be continuous sensations of pleasures and may occur without a climax.

---

[2] Many of these orgasm descriptions were inspired by reading a blog by Annie Sprinkle. As I read, I thought, *Yes, I had that one . . . and that one . . . and that one . . . and then I also experienced some new ones.*

Clitoral Orgasms

These orgasms occur when the clitoris is stimulated and the muscles contract in the vaginal area and then release sexual energy. Clitoral orgasms produce pleasurable sensations that spread through the entire body, from a tingle to a huge contraction that infuses every cell with delight.

Breast/Nipple Orgasms

The breast and nipples are highly sensitive erogenous zones that, when stimulated, produce intensely beautiful orgasms. In sensually heightened moments, the breasts can feel as if they are blossoming with blissful energy, creating a sensation similar to a flower blossoming. Breast and nipple orgasms can be among the strongest because the localized intensity feels like ecstatic love is pouring out of them.

Mouth-to-Throat Orgasms

The lips, mouth, tongue, roof of the mouth, and back of the throat are all erogenous zones. If stimulated in the right way, the throat and thyroid area can actually secrete a fluid much like ejaculation. The ancients called this *amrita*, which means "divine nectar," and it was prized for it healing qualities. After a throat ejaculation you might feel a renewed sense power that allows you to express your truth more easily and authentically. This beautiful experience teaches us that sexual liberation exists beyond our genitals.

Cellular Orgasms

Every time cells multiply in your body, a beautiful release of energy takes place, similar to an orgasm. If you notice, you will feel your cells celebrating their new life. You can also have different orgasmic experiences in your organs; sexual energy can ripple through your lungs, liver, kidneys, and brain. In addition to the mouth and throat, orgasms can also be experienced in your ears and toes. Chills, sneezes, and goosebumps can be transmuted into an orgasm. Even your nervous system can create all sorts of pleasurable bioenergetic responses as its electricity runs through your body!

Pineal Gland Orgasms

Similar to cellular and throat orgasms, the pineal gland can reach high orgasmic states that sometimes ejaculate an *amrita* fluid. The pineal gland is a small, pea-shaped gland in the brain that produces and regulates hormones, including melatonin. It is connected to your crown chakra (your psychic potential) and regulates the serotonin functions that aid sleep and elevate mood. A pineal orgasm can be healing for seekers who wish to awaken their spiritual path and/or train the body to reach heightened vibrational states. The most profound way to experience a pineal gland orgasm is to visualize your sexual energy rising up to stimulate it. At the same time, you can call upon the vibrations of heaven to descend down to it. The upward and downward energies will create a vortex of energy that stimulates the pineal gland to start opening and orgasming with delightful sensations. Imagine a thousand lotus flower petals blossoming to their full glory; the energetic field of your pineal gland will do the same. This process will also indirectly detoxify and strengthen the pineal gland's functions.

Micro-Moment Orgasms

You can experience an orgasm anytime you do an activity that you find pleasurable. It could be anything from walking, singing, sunbathing, dancing under the moonlight, to listening to your favorite music, having a bath, oiling your body, or eating chocolate. These orgasms are created from the sheer joy of what you are experiencing. Bubbling beneath your skin, all you need to do is allow the orgasmic feeling to move through your body and out into your energy field to fall deeper in love with the activity you are doing. These types of orgasms often occur spontaneously, but they can also be taught by adding more loving awareness to your activity.

Breath Orgasms

Breath orgasms can be created through conscious and rhythmical deep breathing as you also intend to move your sexual energy through your body at the same time. Breath orgasms can begin circulating through your body with every inhale and exhale, and then they can extend beyond your body until you feel the divine universe breathing in and out of you. Everything, after all, is expanding and contracting from your lungs to the galaxies.

Emotional Orgasms

These orgasms can occur as a result of intense emotional feelings such as anger, sadness, and amusement (anger-gasms, cry-gasms, laugh-gasms). Have you ever laughed so much that you cried and almost lost your breath? When an intense emotion is experienced, there is also a release of tension. Such a cathartic response can activate an orgasmic release as the body purges the old to welcome the new.

Dream Orgasms

These beautiful orgasms can occur from an erotic and sensual dreams. The dream orgasm becomes a real one, and it can be so intense that it wakes you up. You might feel strong vaginal contractions or subtle vibrations. Dream orgasms not only give us pleasure—they can be healing as well, lingering throughout the day.

Kundalini Orgasms

These orgasms happen when the Kundalini energy begins at the bottom of the spine and travels up through the core of the body, opening up all the chakras to the top of the crown. According to Tantric tradition, Kundalini energy rests like a coiled serpent at the base of the spine. When this dormant energy flows freely upward through the seven chakras, it leads to an expanded state of consciousness known as a Kundalini awakening. The main purpose of Kundalini orgasms is liberating the spirit from the density of the body. In doing so, it can hit against the blocks in the charkas, causing discomfort until the block is released. These orgasms can last anywhere from a minute to several years.

Wave Orgasms

Wave orgasms occur when energy spins through the body creating undulation or wave movements with your arms, legs, spine or body part. Such orgasms have given birth to many of the movements produced in belly dancing. As you move your body, you allow your energy to dip and rise, and this ignites the sexual energy so it can circulate through the body. It also encourages the Kundalini energy at the bottom of the spine to activate.

Heart Orgasms

Heart orgasms are beautiful and do not require any physical stimulation. They can happen while having an inspiring thought that awakens your body to experience love, or when streams of energy pour down from the heavens to align you to your higher purpose. Every higher purpose is an alignment of love, and so in such alignments, the heart center floods open with the ecstatic joy that you have discovered your truth or a revelation has occurred. Heart orgasms can also occur through intention by directing your sexual energy to move up toward the chest and expand through the heart. Focused breathwork can help you achieve this with ease. For instance, on an inhale, squeeze your Kegel muscles (located in your pelvic floor area) and direct your sexual energy up to the heart center. Then on an exhale, direct your sexual energy out the center of your chest. Repeat this a few times while smiling, and you'll begin to notice your heart bubbling with orgasmic sensations.

Life Orgasms

This is when your entire body is one living, breathing, walking, talking orgasm. This usually occurs when you are so deeply in love with life that life itself makes love to you.

Soul Orgasms

Soul orgasms occur when two souls come together to make love, and they synchronize their body, mind, and soul with each other. As their chakras connect, the heart opens, and the benevolent union creates one united orgasm. There is a deep sense of being one with each other, and much soul information can be exchanged. A soul orgasm could be exchanged with your partner for days, weeks, or years. They can occur even if you are not in physical contact with your partner; sometimes the physical distance makes the soul exchange more intense.

Cosmic Orgasms

A cosmic orgasm occurs when there is a cultivation of energy generated by the forces of the cosmos, like the sun or stars, or even through subtle energies such as chi/prana. These orgasms feel as though the sun or the universe is making love to you. Cosmic orgasms can give profound insights and cause an evolution in the physical body. An upgrade of your body and DNA can also occur so that more of your soul and your higher self can exist on Earth.

Rebirth Orgasms

These intense orgasms are felt all over the body, are deeply emotional and, for some, are spiritual and healing experiences. They can last for minutes, hours, or even days. In order to have a rebirth orgasm, you must let go of your identity and be able to handle the voltage of ecstasy that passes through you. A completely purifying and renewing experience, the build-up of old emotions and thoughts is released and replaced by a profound sense of self. It can feel as if you have been birthed by the universe.

Empathetic Orgasms

Empathetic orgasms occur when you are with someone else. When you are in a compassionate space, your body opens up and you can receive the orgasmic waves the other person is emitting from his or her body into yours.

Nature Orgasms

These occur when you are able to pick up and transduce the subtle energies that the trees, flowers, rocks, mountains, souls and crystals emit into orgasms. A beautiful exchange of information and rejuvenation can be given to you by nature.

Divine Orgasms

These occur when the divine vibrations of love that exist through the universe are received by every cell in the body. Like two souls meeting, the vibration of love that exists within you receives the vibrations of love beyond you. From this union, every cell from your toes to your head can orgasm, which opens your body to emit more love to bless life. The painful illusion of divine separation falls away as your body, soul, heart, and mind unites with what it has always longed for. Once a divine orgasm has been experienced, it never ends. Although the intensity may oscillate and at times feel subtle, the divine union that has taken place always remains. A sense of completion and wholeness remains.

My experience in the rainforest was truly multi-orgasmic. It began as a nature orgasm, then continued into a blended orgasm through my genitals, breasts, throat, and cells. The intensity activated my Kundalini energy, which created wave orgasms up and down my spine and opened my heart for a heart, breast, and life orgasm. When those orgasms burst through my pineal gland, my consciousness expanded out into the vast universe. The magical vibrations of the stars and sun activated cosmic orgasms, which opened me up to experience a divine orgasm. I had so many insights, revelations, healings, transmissions, and transformations during each orgasmic moment that my being, my body, and my life was renewed.

Every moment of every day can bring the same sense of renewal—sometimes in profound, mind- and body-blowing ways. Other times we can experience a gentle and delicate renewal that is so subtle that, if you blink, you will miss it. All you need to do is make the choice to relate to your sexual energy as a sacred force. It has the potential to release the love living within your cells, so ecstatic bliss can bounce from your skin to radiate through your aura. You, beautiful woman, live in a very magical body.

Reflection:

1. Reflect upon the vibration of love becoming a physical experience. What does this mean to you?
2. Which part of your body desires to blossom with love the most?
3. What type of orgasms have you already experienced?
4. What orgasms would you like to experience?
5. Can you think of any more types of orgasms not listed?
6. Have you experienced orgasmic energy being blocked in your body?
7. What is the subtlest/smallest orgasms you have experienced? What is the most intense orgasm you have experienced?
8. Close your eyes and tune into your body. Which part naturally feels the most orgasmic?
9. Reflect upon your inner beauty becoming your outer radiance. What difference does this make in your daily life?
10. Explore this cycle: 'opening yourself to receive more love, increases your capacity to love yourself, and this makes you a bigger vessel to receive more love from the universe.'

5

Understanding Your Sacred Sexual Energy

Your sexual energy is key in making the vibration of love an orgasmic and physical experience. It originates as a driving force of nature, from the pollination of plants to the biological urge to reproduce in both animals and humans. Since the human body has the potential to evolve spiritually and energetically, nature has also given sexuality an opportunity to transcend the limits of physical boundaries and elevate you to higher spiritual realms. Sexual energy evolves from the basic need for survival to the altered states of enlightened consciousness, whereby the body, mind, and soul transcend to vibrating strands of loving light.

Your sexual energy exists beyond your genitals; it exists throughout every part of you. It is a life force that pulses and tremors in your cells; it asks you to move and stretch so it can flow more freely. It calls you to transform your limitations so your consciousness can move into freedom.

It does this so you can dance with so much life that a portal of heaven awakens in your body temple.

The sexual energy in your genitals gives you physical power. This could include feelings of sexual arousal, vitality, or a sense that you need to exercise and "burn off" excess energy. When your sexual energy moves up into your heart, it gives you passion, which could include a deep love for yourself, a love for another person, or a deep call to fulfill a desire. As sexual energy travels up toward the head, it takes the heart energy with it, and this fuels your mind to have loving thoughts that are filled with purpose. When your sexual energy travels up to connect to the heavens and out to unite with life, it gives you a sense of position; you are able to claim your right to exist more fully in life. The combination of your sexual energy activating power, passion, purpose, and position centers you in the essence of who you are and what you are here to do. Your sexual energy, when cultivated to move through the chakras, awakens different states of consciousness so your soul can incarnate into your body and fulfill its destiny here on earth—which is ultimately to complete the virtues of love. In order for the vibration of love to exist in the physical world, it needs a body to act from, a heart to feel from, a mind to think from, and a life to live within. Your sexual energy is the fuel that makes all of this happen because it desires to form union and create freedom. It bridges the parts of your awareness that would otherwise exist as separate units and invites them to interact. Your sexual energy is a sacred force that acts like fuel to support and open your body to receive the vibrations of love that exist all around you. A woman's body, mind, heart, and soul need to be nourished by love, and it is your sexual energy which allows this exchange to take place.

In Taoist traditions, sexual energy was trained to move upward for health, vitality, and longevity. The Taoists referred to sexual energy as *jing* - a creative energy vital for the development of *chi* (vital life force energy) and *shen* (spiritual energy). They used sexual energy as a healing force and would direct it into the organs of their body for rejuvenation. Indian tantric traditions also cultivated sexual energy to move upward. Tantric masters understood that when this force was rooted vertically through the body and along the chakras, it could help one move beyond the ego and into oneness. Cultivating your sexual energy to evolve through your body is essential to your spiritual evolution, and it can be achieved through practices without touch or the involvement of another person.

*'Cultivating your sexual energy is essential
for your spiritual evolution.'*

However, many women have been brought up to believe that sexual energy should only be used for procreation or as desire that leads to intimacy with another person. Others have been brought up to believe that they have to hide their sexuality, be ashamed of it, or deny it completely. Our sexual energy often is trapped in a story that inhibits it to exist as a sacred force. Sexual abuse, those in authority shaming you with religious beliefs, partners that may have been unkind during intercourse, or the media objectifying women's sexuality all distort your relationship to your sexual self. Chapter eleven, *The Puzzle Of Love*, will take you deeper into this topic. Your beliefs and experiences either block, inhibit, or arouse sexual energy to flow through your body. Every thought and emotion you experience creates a vibration of energy that ripples through your body to either liberate and open your being to love or contract and disconnect it from love. For this reason, every woman must journey into self-love, where she is able to heal and transform every negative thought, feeling, and perception into love. Self-love is so powerful because it allows you to generate your own love inside your body. This has two effects: first, it helps you become aware that you are a sacred being, and second, your sexual energy is magnetized to love. The more love you generate, the more your sexual energy will become a sacred force which is free to flow through your body and meet the love that exists within and around you.

Liberating Your Female Body

The primary area that a woman feels her sexual energy as a physically arousing force is in and around the vagina. Also known as the *yoni* in Sanskrit – the revered gateway to heaven. Your *yoni* is the sacred portal of your sexual energy and therefore should be honored as your divine inner temple. Many women have forgotten this very sacred part of their body and some of us don't even know what our beautiful flower looks like. Your exquisite *yoni* is the birthplace of life and the origin of all sensual enlightenments. At the end of this chapter you are invited to do *The Sacred Yoni Ritual,* an honoring and activation of the most sacred temple in this universe.

Your sexual energy extends from the *yoni* to the erogenous zones, which stores sexual energy in locations around the body. The main erogenous zones for a woman include her feet, inner thighs, hips, stomach, nipples, upper arms, neck, lips, mouth, ears, and head. This, of course, does not exclude other body parts, and each woman has a unique blueprint of where her sensitivity is located. Remember, sexual energy seeks freedom, so any part of your being that experiences a sense of liberating energy passing through is due to your sexual energy. Depending on the libido, some women experience their sexual energy as a strong, pulsing feeling. Some feel it like ripples of energy passing through their body, while others experience it as localized pleasure. And in many women, it's a dormant energy waiting to be aroused.

The key is to become more conscious of the sexual energy blossoming through your body. Smile when you notice it, because it's such a beautiful part of you. Next, allow it to have the freedom to move through your body anywhere it likes. Dancing is a wonderful way to aid and celebrate the sexual energy traveling through your body. Many of the undulating movements belly dancers make are created to allow the sexual energy to travel like a wave up though the hips, spine, and arms. Your sexual energy can also be stimulated through touch, movement, deep breathing, optimum hormonal health, sexual intimacy with another, a fantasy, a dream, a desire, a spiritual awakening, an arousing thought, and proper nutrition and exercise. Everybody's sexual energy gets stimulated differently; the key is to let it travel through the body so you can feel your sexual energy making love to more of you. Your sexual energy can be stimulated to awaken anytime and anywhere. It might happen in the supermarket, while you are going for a walk, taking a shower, going to the toilet, eating an apple, or singing a song. Sexual awakenings are not confined to the bedroom, nor are they dependent on anyone else. They are simply bursts of ecstatic joy that have freedom to move through your body.

'Sexual awakenings are not confined to the bedroom, nor are they dependent on anyone else.'

Kundalini

As mentioned in the previous chapter, at the base of your spine is another great storehouse of sexual energy known as the Kundalini. *Kundalini* is a Sanskrit word that translates as "coiled one," and it describes the primal energy that helps one awaken to higher spiritual awareness. This energy spirals from the base of the spine to the crown of the head, opening and clearing the chakras as it moves up - liberating and transforming the limited egoic self into the true nature as a divine being. Some refer to this as the Kundalini Shakti, because Shakti is that which has materialized from the heaven energy. In Hindu culture Shakti is the personification of the divine feminine that represents the creative power within everything to manifest the divine into physical form. Your journey into sensual enlightenment also aims to help you birth your divine soul into your physical body. The Kundalini energy sits at the base of the spine like a coiled snake, and when activated, it rises through the central *nadi*, an energy pathway running through the central core of the body. It also can be felt either inside or alongside the spine, moving though the body like electric energy to the top to the head. As the Kundalini moves up, it activates the seven chakras that are located through the body. When the Kundalini progresses through each chakra, a different awakening or mystical experience can occur, until it reaches the crown where a profound transformation of consciousness can take place.

Such experiences bring deep states of enlightenment, feelings of bliss, infinite love, and universal connectivity. On a physical level, rushes of energy, heightened sensations, shaking, tingling, involuntary jerks, and intense heat or cold can be felt throughout the body as it awakens to becoming a higher vibration of love.

Kundalini energy is a very powerful force that is needed to open the energy pathways that would otherwise remain blocked. The more energy pathways you have flowing with your sexual energy, the more conscious and alive you will feel. As the Kundalini energy opens each of the charkas, a lot of old emotions and karmic baggage that have clogged the energy in your body are released. This can sometimes create headaches or pressure inside the body. Often these blocks require healing assistance or deep reflection to help them transform. Kundalini rising can range from intense experiences to those that are very subtle, and they can last for a few minutes to days or even years. The key is knowing how to transform the energy blocks so it can be a comfortable experience. The ultimate aim of the game is to unlock those blocks with self-love so you can liberate your energy to keep ascending. This process of transforming the limitations within generates much insight about love and the truth of who you are authentically. Every lotus must rise from her mud, and the kundalini awakenings are designed to do this. How else will you blossom into the beautiful being that you truly are? Chapter Eight, *The Lotus Transcends from Her Mud*, will teach you how to release your blocks.

Sexual Life Force Ascends through the Chakras

As your sexual life forces ascend up your body and pass through each chakra, fresh awareness awakens, and this empowers you to exist as an authentic individual. Remember, your sexual energy acts as a strengthening force so the love within you has a firm foundation from which to exist. As your sexual energy supports your base chakra, you begin to feel secure in your body, and this will then support your sacral chakra to feel safe enough to exist in sensual freedom. As your sexual energy continues to rise, it will shine out of your solar plexus and give you the power to say yes or no and absolutely mean it. When you heart blossoms with sexual energy, the infinite pool of love that exists within you finally has the fuel to radiate out into your life. This will warm your heart and your body with so much contentment that your deep loneliness will disappear. The sexual energy in your heart will teach you to honor, respect, and be proud of the unique individual you are.

In the ecstatic knowing that more of your uniqueness can exist, your heart pushes your sexual energy to your throat chakra, giving you the strength and the conviction to express your truth at all times. As your sexual energy continues to rise, it empowers your mind to have clearer thoughts. Making decisions will be easier, and you will stop collapsing into negative or anxious thinking. The sexual energy will continue to ascend, connecting the crown of your head to the heavens above and merging your sense of identity with life. This activates your intuitive senses and opens your being to receive profound insights about life and your life purpose. Your sexual energy's role is to activate your chakras so more of your consciousness can exist in physical reality. Your sexual energy will strengthen each chakra so that it can support the chakra above to open. This will then help unite all of your chakras to operate as one force so your unique identity can shine with presence. In order to help the process of your sexual energy ascending up the body, one very important ingredient is required, and that is Earth energy.

'Your sexual energy needs the earth's energy to support it.'

Sexual Energy Activators

The Earth has its own sexual energy that rises up from the ground, known as the Earth Shakti. This beautiful force makes trees, flowers, and your body grow tall. Your sexual energy needs the Earth's energy to support it. Just as trees have roots to get nourishment from the Earth, all the energy pathways in your body, particularly in your feet, can also be rooted into the ground and drink up the earth's energy to nourish the body. The Earth's Shakti supports your sexual energy, and the more you allow your body to be fed by the earth, the more content, grounded, and present you will feel. Much of the loneliness we feel is actually caused by a disconnect from the Earth. You must learn to be supported by it.

It was only when my awakening in the rainforest occurred, that I discovered my sexual energy was a sacred force that could strengthen, and rejuvenate my entire being. Before that I just thought it was meant to be given away in relationships. I spent years longing for someone else to complete me with their energy, but it wasn't until my sexual energy got activated by the earth's energy that my whole perception changed. My sexual energy was no longer something I exchanged for intimacy, but rather a life force that could rejuvenate me body, mind, heart, and soul. As the earth pushed my sexual energy up through my body, it opened my chakras and pushed my essence through each one. As it did, I immediately began to experience the positive function each chakra had, and this made me feel powerful, beautiful, and in command of my life. My sexual energy brought new life to the parts of my body that had been closed and dormant. It made me present with my sense of self from my head to my toes. No longer lost inside and disconnected, my sexual energy somehow stitched my soul through my energy pathways and chakras so I could exist in my body. The more present I became in my body, the more I could feel myself glowing with my own soul light. My thoughts became clearer with my truth, and I felt a power that rang all the way down to my bones and all the way through my energy field. I felt like a warrior queen who was completely in command of everything in her own unique reality. This was the female empowerment I had always wanted to embody, and I am in deep gratitude for the energy of Mother Nature to initiate this awakening.

That being said, particular sacred sites around our planet—special waterfalls, caves, mountains, nature spots like the Daintree Rainforest, and temples— have special openings that allow more of the Earth's energy to pass through. If you visit one of these significant sites, you often will experience a transference of powerful energy. The Kundalini within the spine gets activated and a special awakening occurs. The sun, moon, stars, planets, and all the cosmic energy in the universe also have the potential to charge your sexual energy like a battery. Just as you have energy pathways that go down into the earth, they also extend up into the sky to receive cosmic energies. You are a part of everything in this universe, and your body requires nourishment from different sources. The inner hunger you feel is often because you have not learned how to be nourished by the forces of nature that surround you.

Your sexual energy loves to experience connection and intimacy, and it longs to unite with the different life forces existing within and around you. This creates a cocktail of energies, that are always mixing and meeting each other inside your body. Your loving sexual energy fuses it all together to generate a new experience. It is in this process that orgasms are experienced, insights are generated, and new energies are created. The experience of sexual energy uniting with the heart, is a different experience from the sexual energy uniting with the mind, or some other organ. It is different again when your sexual energy unites with the stars or sun. From every star in the sky to every grain of sand, every cell in your body is meant to energetically feel connected to life, and your sexual energy is the catalyst to make this happen. Your body temple is the melting pot for all of these energies, and through the virtues of love—relating, exchanging, desiring, connecting, and being intimate with these forces—the dynamic experiences of love gets created. This is how you make love to yourself, make love to life, and allow life to make love to you. When all your energy connects to all of life and beyond, you feel a deep oneness with the universe.

Your sexual energy is also charged by other people's sexual energy. Man or woman, everyone's sexual energy is uniquely coded with information that can activate and awaken us. The key is to choose the partners who will raise you into an experience of love and hold you through whatever process of lovemaking is required to achieve this, and vice versa. When this occurs, your partner's sexual energy enters into your body and ignites your sexual energy. If your partner connects to you in love, all of his or her information of love will enter into your body to educate you, and vice versa. Lovemaking is a beautiful exchange where sexual energy and love unite, explode, enliven, and encode both partners to become better. On the flip side, if your partner is unable to hold you in a space of love, intimate experiences may leave you feeling drained, deflated, confused, or numb. This is because love has not been generated and the exchange of information has not taken place. In worst cases, one partner could drain the life force of the other to supply their own needs. Sometimes both partners do this, leading to quite toxic relationships.

When I was in my early twenties, I experienced a similar relationship. In the beginning we were totally infatuated with each other. There was passion, romance, intimacy, and a magnetic spark that kept pulling us together. Unfortunately, he had an addictive personality; he smoked and drank, and eventually I became his addiction as well. At first it was wonderful to get so much attention, but then he constantly wanted me, and I felt drained every time I left him. I had no time to see friends or study, and I began to put on weight as a form of protection. It was only when he said, "I need you so I can be happy," that I realized the type of relationship I was in. Our breakup was difficult, and he threatened to commit suicide if I left him. Nonetheless I did, and within a month I naturally lost all the weight I put on, my energy returned, and I felt like my life and body belonged to me again. This relationship taught me to recognize the difference between healthy and needy intimate exchanges, and I became aware that I should only give my energy to those who are able to share theirs with me in a healthy way. I learned that my sexual life force is a precious commodity.

Scaffolding for Your Soul

You have thousands of energy pathways in your body, and your sexual energy is designed to flow through them to help fortify your body. Just as scaffolding supports a building, your sexual energy strengthens your body and your auric field. The stronger your physical and energy bodies are with your sexual life force, the more your soul can integrate into your body.

Your soul—which some refer to as your higher self—is the part of you that comes from love. You soul is like a drop in the ocean of love and it holds the wisdom you need to navigate through life. The more present your soul is in your body, the more mastery you will have over your life. Your soul's destiny is to create love in your life. Through the journey of self-love, you can expand from being an individual to being one with all of existence. When your sexual energy extends into your energy field, more love and more of your soul can exist within and around your body. As your sexual energy continues to expand up to the heavens and out into life, your energy field grows larger and larger, calling more love and more of your soul to incarnate into your body. It does this by activating the energy pathways through and beyond your body, creating a bridge for your soul's energy to merge and integrate back into your physical cells. As the soul vibration unites with the body, it is energized by its higher purpose. Creative energy then flows through the body, inspiring you to take physical action so your destiny can be realized. Many of the impulsive desires you have—such as going to a particular concert or café, reading a particular book, talking to a particular person, or traveling to a specific country—is the sublimation of your sexual energy willing your soul's destiny into physical reality. This "all-body impulse" is often your soul rerouting you so that you meet the people you are meant to meet and do the things you are meant to do to master your life.

In the peak of such experiences, an intensity of energy is created in the body as love tries to give birth through the cells. Such experiences offer a rebirth into a more refined version of yourself plus a cellular shift into a higher vibrational realm of love. This can be a very cathartic experience, leaving one changed forever and often with a new life path or direction. Sensual enlightenment occurs because, as a woman, you have the ability to rebirth your entire body into a more sublime frequency of love—again and again and again. Through this reconnection, a deep fulfilment of love is experienced, where the excess of love's vibration that you have accumulated in your cells will overflow and shine out to bless life. This is what gives you the potential to be a portal of love.

'Your sexual energy will sublimate into spiritual energy.'

Once the sexual energy is freed to exist as a sacred force that is experiencing love, the sexual energy will sublimate into spiritual energy.

Spiritual energy is made up of the higher frequencies of love, and it brings ecstatic awakening and profound insights. Your sexual energy is a highly arousing force. On a physical level it activates the body and the senses to experience orgasms. As your sexual energy transcends into spiritual energy, your five senses (touch, taste, hearing, sight, smell) evolve into psychic senses—clairvoyance, clairsentience, clairaudience, empathic sense, and prophetic sense—which then are able to create ecstatic epiphanies and sensual enlightenment. The experiences a woman can have with her sexual energy are infinite: from multidimensional intuitive experiences to multiorgasmic physical experiences. When these states combine, the totality of love's thirteen virtues can be experienced at once, granting you the guiding force to navigate and recreate your life.

My awakening in the rainforest was a destined moment for me for two reason: it prepared my body for my daughter and it initiated my journey into sensual enlightenment. At the peak of the experience when my sexual energy sublimated through my body to connect my consciousness to the heavens, a download of awareness entered my body and activated my cells to function in a new way. In this moment I was able to transduce the universal field of love through my body, and as a result, my mind, heart, and senses opened to transmit it into the physical world. My body channeled it orgasmically, but the rest of my being translated the energy of love as an awareness that brought wisdom, passion, union, creation, desire, power, wonder, and joy all at once. In that moment, my being experienced the virtues of love simultaneously, and my vibration transcended until I felt one with both life and love. This profound union reeducated my concept of reality and rewired my body to function in a new way.

The energy of my awakening continues to flow through me and bring new purpose to my life. From it I have created books, online courses, meditations, retreats, and workshops. It expresses itself in my relationships, as I mother my daughter and teach my students. It still ripples through my body, bringing delight and sensuality in small ways and in big ways. Through certain sensual blossoming exercises, I can sublimated my sexual energy through my body and be made love to by the universe at will. My awakening changed the trajectory of my life, and I hope it changes yours.

Supporting Your Sexual Energy

The fluctuating hormones of the menstrual cycle can also make the physical experience of sexual energy change just like the seasons. The spring of your sexual energy can feel like a bubbling beauty that wants to blossom with new life. The summer of your sexual energy can be fiery, filled with passion and desire for another. The autumn of your sexual energy may feel like you need to return to yourself and focus on self-care. The winter of your sexual energy may feel nonexistent and therefore gives you the space to experience rebirth with new needs. The beauty of seasons is that they are always changing, so embrace the cycles that your sexual energy brings. Each one will teach you something valuable about yourself. Always listen to the changing needs of your sexual energy on emotional, physical and spiritual levels.

You can also support your sexual energy through the foods you choose to eat (and not eat). Reducing foods that disrupt your hormones and lower your immunity and energy levels is essential. Instead of excessive amounts of meat, dairy, alcohol, coffee, and white carbohydrates, you can choose to focus on foods that boost your circulation, energy levels, and regulate your hormones and body sensitivity. An all-natural diet rich in aphrodisiac foods and herbs is best. Bananas are high in potassium and increase the muscle strength needed to pump sexual energy through the body. Pomegranates, known as love apples, are high in antioxidants and increases the blood flow needed to heighten sensitivity. Celery is filled with androgens (a group of hormones similar to testosterone) and have been known to increase libido, particularly in women. Spicy foods such as chili gets your heart pumping, stimulates nerve endings, and increases blood flow. Oysters are high in zinc and help regulate the hormones. Chocolate contains nutrients that increase serotonin levels and boost mood levels. Many herbs can boost your libido, including maca, ginseng, tribulus, and red clover. These herbs are known as adaptogens, meaning they will stimulant your sexual energy and support your hormones and endocrine systems. Herbs are very powerful, so depending on your body's needs, it is important to consult a trained herbalist or nutritionist to choose the ones that are best for you.

Reclaiming Your Sexual Self

Reclaiming your sexual self is one of the most important initiations you can do for yourself as a woman. It is an essential requirement for traveling the path of sensual enlightenment. Your sexual energy is a potent and powerful force, and it belongs solely to you. No longer can you leave the exclusive responsibility of your sexual satisfaction and sexual evolution to your partner. Relying on someone else to make you feel loved, cherished, or liberated is a road that will ultimately leave you feeling dissatisfied. Dissatisfaction turns into disappointment and then loneliness. Two things happen from here: either you begin to disconnect from your partner, or you begin looking for someone else to satisfy and complete you. But this is a myth, for only you can truly complete your wholeness. The power is not outside of you but inside.

When you claim your sexual energy as a sacred force, you no longer leak it or give it away. You stop attracting relationships that dishonor your sacredness. You remove yourself from situations that drain your spirit, and you no longer give in to the media culture where sex is advertised as a cheap commodity. Once you claim your sexual energy as your own, you acknowledge yourself as precious. Precious by definition means "valuable, greatly loved, and treasured," and this is what you are—precious.

Reclaiming your sexual energy as a sacred force within is the first step to harnessing and cultivating its spiritual powers. Your sexual energy is a divine force, and when it is allowed to flow through your body, it will give you a glow, make you feel radiant, and put the spring back in your step. It will become the physical energy needed to manifest your dreams in physical reality, as well as the magnetic energy used to attract goodness into your life.

One of my daily practices is to allow my sexual energy the freedom to light up my inner beauty. I particularly like to do it while walking down the street or while in the supermarket. As I let myself shine with all of who I am, I feel more beautiful and radiant. People around me notice it, and I smile more because my presence makes them feel brighter. Others move out of my way because they feel my energy setting stronger boundaries, and at the same time I get more compliments. When I allow my sexual energy to enliven my presence, I experience a deep sense of contentment, no longer needing, no longer hungry—just the joy that

I exist. My senses heighten; music sounds more vibrant, and smells are more fragrant. As I turn myself on, the life around me turns on as well.

Your beautiful body is built to experience your sexual energy as a spiritual experience on a physical, emotional, mental, spiritual, soul, and evolutionary level. As a result, your sexual energy can be used to create, heal and transform your life. All you need to do is claim it as a sacred force, and no one but you can do this.

Sacred Body Ritual

The best way to claim your sexual energy as a sacred force is perform a ritual that honors it as such. Start by becoming as naked as you feel comfortable so that you can connect and commune with your body temple. You entered into this world naked, so this ritual also acts as a rebirth. Set an intention: what do you wish to rebirth into? Create a sacred space and remove all distractions for at least an hour. You can set an alarm if you feel it will help you relax more deeply into the process and avoid stress if you have other things to do. The key is to do the following actions with reverence. This, after all, is a ceremony to honor your beautiful self's sexual energy. An easy way to do this is to go through all of the actions first in your mind. That way, when you are ready to do them, awareness has already been created.

1. Create your sacred space. Light some candles, put on relaxing music, fill the air with beautiful aromas, and have a nice cushion or pillow to sit on.
2. Sit in your sacred space and breathe deeply. Place your hands on your heart and smile; this initiates the beginning of the ritual. Then like a prayer, say your rebirth intention out loud. Let the vibrations of those words ripple through your body, cells, and soul. Smile and allow your new self to awaken.
3. Begin by stroking your beautiful skin. As you do, smile and feel love for those body parts.
4. Continue this process, each time removing a layer of clothing. Take your time. You are here to ensure that your body feels precious. As you progress through this ritual, you may notice a variety of feelings arising inside. Some body parts may feel forgotten, or sad. Other

body parts may feel excited and joyful. Just witness the feelings that surface and smile into any parts that don't feel so great.

5. When you are as naked as you feel comfortable, allow your hands to dance and glide all over your skin. You may like to use scented oil or natural body lotion. If you do, take the time to smell the fragrance. The key here is to feel gratitude and love for your body. This is your time to fall in love with your body, especially the parts which you have not always loved. You can say affirmations like "I love you"; "I am grateful for my body"; "My body brings joy"; "My body allows me to live." Be open to kind words flowing from your soul, out of your mouth, and into your body. Do this step for as long as you can. Sometimes it takes a little time to warm up, but keep going until you feel yourself flowing.

6. Place your hands over your womb space and, with intention, contact your sexual energy and just allow it to exist. Smile as you feel it rising and bubbling within. If you like, you can practice inviting your sexual energy up through your body on each inhale. Then on each exhale, allow your sexual energy to blossom through the cells of your body. You'll begin to feel as if you are shinning after this practice.

7. Now either stand or kneel. Take your favorite essential oil to anoint your chakras. Focus on each chakra, and as you do, inhale your sexual energy up to that chakra. As you exhale, direct your sexual energy through that chakra to open and activate it. Put a new drop of oil on each chakra as you progress through the ritual. You may want to say:

8. BASE: "I welcome my sexual energy to support into my life." With gratitude, breathe in the blessing of support.

9. SACRAL: "I welcome my sexual energy to bring pleasure into my life." With gratitude, breathe in the blessing of pleasure.

10. SOLAR: "I welcome my sexual energy to make me feel beautiful." With gratitude, breathe in the blessing of beauty.

11. HEART: "I welcome my sexual energy to awaken love into my body and my life." With gratitude, breathe in the blessing of love.

12. THROAT: "I welcome my sexual energy to activate my truth and expression." With gratitude, breathe in the blessing of sacred truth.

13. BROW: "I welcome my sexual energy to activate my intuition and divine wisdom." With gratitude, breathe in the blessing of intuition and divine wisdom.
14. CROWN: "I welcome my sexual energy to activate divinity in all areas of my life." With gratitude, breathe in the blessing of divinity
15. Rub your oiled hands together, brush the fragrance over your body, and celebrate your sexual energy as a sacred force that glows through you.
16. When you feel complete, place your hands on your heart, breathe, smile, and feel the love that has been generated by your body. Stay in that place for a couple of minutes.
17. Place your hands on the ground, then anchor your new awareness through your body and into the earth.
18. Finish with your hands in a prayer position.

Sacred Yoni Ritual

This ritual is a very special ceremony. It initiates your vagina to become the most sacred spot, in the most sacred temple, in the most sacred universe. Create a sacred space and eliminate distractions for at least 2 hours. One hour for the ceremony and another hour to integrate the initiation in a peaceful environment. Light candles, scent the room, choose relaxing music, prepare and oil your beautiful body. It is suggested that you be completely naked for this ritual. You will need 6 candles to represent heaven, 6 pink flowers or crystals to represent love, and 6 leaves or pebbles to represent the earth. If you can, choose to sit in the centre of the room, with space all around you. This represents the centre of the universe.

1. Begin the ritual standing up. Stretch your hands up into the heavens and channel divine energy through your body and into the earth. Spin around in a circle, allowing your body to spiral heaven down to the ground.
2. Once you have energised your body. Place your hands above your womb in the Shakti mudra position and say, 'I am the most sacred spot, in the most sacred temple, in the most sacred universe.' Repeat this several times until your body glows.

3. Take the candles and place them around you. Light them and say 'My inner temple is divine.' 'My inner temple is heaven.' 'My inner temple is sacred.' Continue saying these affirmations until all the candles are lit.

4. Kneel down and sit comfortably in this sacred ring of fire. With intention draw a sacred circle connecting the candles together. Feel your inner temple protected. Meditate for a while and acknowledge the sacredness of your inner temple.

5. Now take the pink flowers or crystals and place them in a circle around you too. If it feels right place the pink flowers or crystals on the outside of the candles. As you place them down say, 'Only love enters.' 'Only love enters.' Continue saying these affirmations until all flowers or crystals are placed down. Place one hand on your heart and one hand on your womb. Meditate for a while and acknowledge what it feels like when only love enters your inner temple.

6. Take the leaves or pebbles and place them around in the circle. As you do say 'I have a voice.' 'I have a choice.' 'My outer temple is cared for.' 'My inner temple is respected.' Continue saying these affirmations until all the leaves or pebbles are laid down. Perhaps you could say an affirmation about how you would like your partner to treat your inner temple. Meditate for a while and acknowledge the respect that your inner temple deserves.

7. Spend some time lovingly caressing every inch of your body until you glow with self love. You may like to use body oil.

8. Place both hands over your *yoni* and feel the power that exists there. Visualise your *yoni* in the centre of the universe with creation energy flowing out of it. Allow your yoni to shine its magical light into your room and out into the world.

9. Then say, 'I am a Goddess.' 'I am a Goddess.' 'I am a Goddess.' Or whatever other power words you would like to use.

10. Meditate on your sacred inner temple for as long as you like.

11. Gently blow out the candles when you are ready to finish.

* Both of these rituals come from my *Sensual Enlightenment Online Academy*. If you would like to unlock the magic of your female body temple then visit www.vanyasilverten.com for more details.

Reflection:

1. Why is it important to let your sexual energy move up through your body?
2. In what circumstances have you have given away your sexual life force to another and felt worse afterward?
3. In what circumstances have you shared your sexual life force with another and have felt brighter?
4. Have you experienced your energy activating from a sacred site? From a person? Or from the cosmos?
5. What is your connection to the earth energy? Do you feel connected to it? Or do you feel separate from the earth? What can you do to help the earth energies support your body more?
6. What foods do you need to eliminate from your diet to increase your sexual energy?
7. What foods do you need to eat in order to increase your sexual energy?
8. What kind of physical exercise will support your body?
9. What does 'claiming your sexual energy as a sacred force' mean to you?
10. If your sexual energy evolves to becoming a sacred force, how will it improve your relationship to your body, your relationships, and your life?
11. How did the *Sacred Yoni Ritual* make you feel?

6

The Art of Blossoming

Sexual energy is magnetized to the vibration of love. In order for the human body to spiritually evolve, it must train the sexual life force to move toward the heart and the heavens. Your sexual energy helps you to flower love through every cell, every organ, and every chakra so you can have a total body experience of love. Your sexual energy offers the physical energy, to support the waves of orgasmic love, that pass through you. Through this process millions of energy pathways are created, and this allows you to refine your body and consciousness, to the high vibrations of love. Just like scaffolding supports a structure as it gets built, your sexual energy offers the same support to your energy field. This is so your soul can expand indefinitely and multidimensionally into love. This awakening never ends. All you need to do is aid the ecstatic vibration of love within you, to blossom and meet the vibration of love outside of you. The art of blossoming refers to the process of how a woman births love from the heavens, through her body, and then shines it out to awaken life.

Your exquisite female body is waiting to bloom. Encoded within every cell of your body, is the awareness that the vibration of love, must blossom through your mind, heart, breasts, and vagina. You are designed to flower this love through your body, and as this occurs, it releases the lower vibrations that clog your cells and energy pathways. Every time your being awakens with the consciousness of love, an enlightenment occurs, your vibration increases, and you are moved into a higher dimension of reality. Old perceptions are liberated into new ones, limited beliefs and outdated paradigms are transformed, and you align to who you authentically are. When you upgrade your worldview, you no longer act from judgment or defensiveness, and this helps you to act with more compassion. Such blossomings, can gift you with heightened insights and feelings of love that rush through your body - awakening every cell with new awareness. You, beautiful woman, are designed to flower with ecstatic revelations, of how to proceed forward as an empowered woman.

'Your female body is designed to blossom with love.'

Your ability to witness love manifesting into reality makes you a creator of love. This is why you may feel you live in a world that does not make sense to you. When life does not reflect love, it can make you feel sad, withdrawn, shut down, scared, anxious, or just very disappointed. All of these reactions make you feel powerless, but this is not your truth. The truth is that you have been designed to blossom with the power and beauty of love; you have been created to heal and transform everything within and around you. When you remember how the exquisite mechanics of your female body operate, you will discover how easy it is to transcend any corrupted versions of reality. This is your true power and your true beauty.

The art of blossoming is an essential requirement to experience sensual enlightenment. It is only through your body that the physical experience of love can manifest. Without your body, love remains merely a vibration, and heaven just a concept. Your task is to cultivate and train your sexual energy, and as you do, you will notice that a youthful glow will return to your skin, and your body will have a fresh vibrancy. The art of blossoming is the perfect antiaging remedy! All you have to do is practice it.

The Blossoming Essentials

Before we progress to the movements that cause love to blossom through your body, your practice begins with embodying six foundation exercises: breath, movement, smiling, touch, sounding, and shining. Each of these will activate your sexual energy - turning it into a sacred fuel for your body.

1. Breath

Breath is essential to your life. Breathing deeply and evenly fuels your body with oxygen, the much-needed nutrient that energizes your cells. The air you breathe is filled with prana, the universal life force that vitalizes all matter. On occasion you may notice gold strands of light dancing through the air. This is prana, and your body ingests it through your breath. The key to breathing, is to breathe all the way down to your belly, and completely fill your lungs with new air. This will charge your body like a battery. Many of us are shallow breathers and are not used to having an adequate supply of oxygen. Deep and conscious breathing may make you feel dizzy at first, but as you practice, your body will get used to being energized by oxygen. After you've learned to breathe deeply, you can advance this process by intending every cell in your body to breathe in prana as well. This is as simple as visualizing each of your cells with a mouth, and then intend each of your cells to inhale and exhale, as you inhale and exhale. This process will energize your body to become a super battery of vibrancy.

2. Movement

Your sexual energy depends upon your muscles to move it through your body. Your muscles act like a pump, and with every contraction and relaxation, you can direct your sexual energy to transcend. The undulation movements in belly dancing are examples of this. The hips, belly, and arms move like waves to the eye, but physically it begins first with one area of the muscles contracting and releasing. This then brings energy to the muscles above, which continue the process of moving energy by contracting and releasing, to the next set of muscles. Just like a snake ripples its body as it moves, you can do the same, and as you do, sexual energy moves from the genitals up toward the arms and head. This same principle applies to the delicate muscles in the vaginal area, that help both to stimulate and direct, the sexual energy throughout the body.

3. Smiling

Smiling is essential to create joy inside your body. Every time you smile you activate serotonin levels in the brain and balance hormones in the body. Each smile stimulates the heart chakra to open and radiate love to fuel the energy pathways in your body. Just as every cell in your body can breathe in prana, likewise every cell in your body can smile. Intending every cell in your body to smile stimulates the love within you to shine out. Allowing your entire body to smile brings contentment; your anxieties will subside, and your beauty will glow.

4. Touch

Touch is a beautiful act of affection and self-love. Every time you touch your skin, you stimulate the energy pathways in your body to start flowing. Begin by caressing the curves of your body toward your heart center; this promotes the physical experience of self-love, which is very warming for the body. Next, focusing your touch on your erogenous zones, stimulates the sexual energy stored within and allows it to blossom. You will feel your sensual beauty moving from inside to outside your body.

5. Sound

You voice is a powerful tool that expresses your inner world to the outer world. A powerful woman is one who can voice her truth. Learning to vocalize the beauty that exists within, helps you to become more confident in your sense of self. First it begins as tones, then progresses to orgasmic sounds, and if you release all inhibition, you may even belt out the song of your soul. Practice making a tone with every breath you exhale, then progress to sounding the pleasure that moves through your body when you exhale.

6. *Shining*

Shinning occurs when your entire being glows with your unique vibration. Through intention, every cell in your body can glow like the sun. All you have to do is focus on the light that exists inside of you and will it to shine. Allowing your body to shine raises your sense of self-esteem and helps you to feel proud of who you are. It is your sexual energy and the love inside your cells that make you glow. All you have to do is cultivate those two forces inside of you.

> *'It is your sexual energy and the love inside your cells that make you glow.'*

Eventually all of these foundation exercises come together like an improvised dance. Your deep breathing combined with touch, will activate the love in your cells and energize the sexual energy in your body. Your muscles will direct your beautiful essence around your body, and with an immense feeling of self-love, you will naturally desire to make your inner beauty shine out into the world as radiance. You celebrate the whole process with your voice, letting it sound out the experience of your body blossoming its sensual pleasure.

The Blossoming Movements Bring Awareness

As you practice the six foundation exercises, you will then be able to use your consciousness to take your body to the next level. Blossoming love through your body, via your sexual energy, is a movement that unfolds within you just like petals opening to the sun. Each movement is designed to bring awareness to your body - teaching you how to consciously cultivate your sexual energy, so more love can flower through you. Each of these movements are ordered so you can become aware of the layers of energy existing within you. However, each movement can occur spontaneously at any time, and all movements can occur at once, when the body is able to filter everything through the vibration of love. To help heighten the experience, please visualize and feel each of the steps, becoming as conscious as you can of the energy moving through you. The more you practice the movement exercises, the more your awareness will develop to experience sensual enlightenments. Please refer to the key so that you can decode the supporting images.

The Key

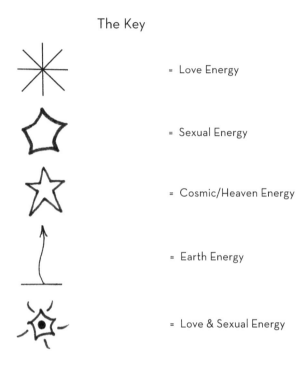

= Love Energy

= Sexual Energy

= Cosmic/Heaven Energy

= Earth Energy

= Love & Sexual Energy

Awareness 1: Love Is All Around You

The vibration of love exists all around you. It exists in the space between every atom and molecule, and it also exists within every atom and molecule that has chosen to manifest love into reality. When you acknowledge that you come from and live within the vibration of love, something very magical happens. Each of your five senses, plus every cell in your body, seeks to unite and connect with both its manifested and unmanifested forms. The manifested forms of love can come from the kindness of other people, lovemaking, smelling a rose, feeling the sun on your skin, tasting a juicy piece of fruit, or beautiful memories surfacing to make you smile.

Unmanifested forms of love are revealed through insights, apparitions of angels or ascended masters, or high vibrational energies transmitting from the field of love into the body. Love comes in many forms, but it is only though the body that enlightenment can be a multidimensional sensual experience. From the heavens to the earth, love will manifest itself. It is through your developed senses that you will be able translate the spectrum of experience love transmits. All you have to do is learn to discern what comes from love and what doesn't. As a woman, you train your senses to be able to decipher the truth in every micro-moment. Not every person or experience offers love. Sometimes our desperate need to be loved or experience love can skew our perceptions, and we can get caught in an illusion. That's why it is of the utmost importance that you honor the journey of self-love so you can, refine and direct your inner compass to love. When you choose to live in a reality that vibrates with love, miracles and synchronicities manifest more easily. Divine timings and chance meetings become the norm because, love itself is constantly presenting scenarios to help you evolve into the greatest version of yourself. In this awareness you are always being supported, guided, and nourished by love itself.

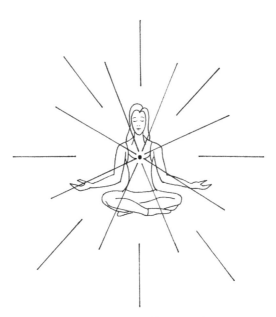

Figure 1: Love Is All Around You

Movement Exercise - *refer to figure 1:*

1. One of the simplest ways to perceive the great field of love that surrounds you, is to sit very quietly - calming your body and mind with deep breaths. Once you feel your awareness drop into your heart, you will begin to feel your heart chakra relaxing and expanding. As you keep breathing your awareness through your heart center, allow your energy body to expand.

2. On every exhale, you expand your energy, while on every inhale you open your energy body and breathe in the vibration of love. The vibration of love is easy to find if you notice the space between the atoms that surround you. Everything that looks solid around you is actually vibrating. The walls, the doors, and the trees are all pulsing with energy, just like your body. When you expand your energy body into the space that exists within everything, you will notice love's vibration shining and smiling at you.

3. Once you feel this ecstatic frequency - on the inhale breathe love back into your heart and then exhale that love through your body to nourish every cell. If you like, visualize every cell in your body having a mouth that can drink in love. Repeat this a few times.

4. Next bring your awareness into every cell and on the inhale, visualize each cell breathing in the great vibration of love back into your body. On the exhale, allow every cell in your body to breathe love back out to bless life.

5. Repeat this a few times until your feel united with love. This exercise teaches, that you can unite with the great field of love at will. The key is to never feel disconnected from it, and to recognize that the connection is only an intention away.

Awareness 2: Love Is Within You

Your origin is love and every single cell in your body is coded with love. When you decided to incarnate into your body, you brought the vibration of love with you. From the moment of conception, you chose to imprint every atom and molecule that formed you with love. You may have been born into a family that had distorted genetics and corrupted understandings of love, and that may have confused your thoughts and feelings. But nonetheless you come from love, and the "mud" your family gave you becomes a blessing when you flower out of it. Since every cell in your body comes from love, every cell is also coded to blossom with love. Love only knows how to expand and grow. It is an act of self love to notice and will more love to exists inside of you. The love that comes from your cells is infinite; it does not end because that love flows from the great field of love. Every cell in your body is a gateway and turns into a chakra when love emits from it. A chakra is a spinning vortex of energy, and since you have billions of cells, you also have billions of chakras. The endless supply of love within you means that you have enough fuel to love every organ in your body back to health, transform every negative thought, and raise the world around you into a higher frequency of love. Your ability to radiate love gives you presence. This presence makes people notice you because you change the energy of the environment wherever you go. The ability to transmit love from your cells, to connect to the vibration of love that exists everywhere, completes a very important circuit. In fact, it is probably the most important circuit that your body will ever make, without it the rest of your path into sensual enlightenment will not happen. It is this circuit where the internal love vibration and the external love vibration meet.

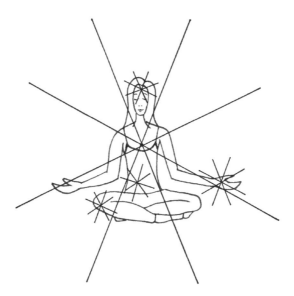

Figure 2: Love Is Within You

Movement Exercise - *refer to figure 2:*

1. Take a few deep breaths and become more and more relaxed in your body. Let you mind calm and your heart open. As you notice every cell in your body shining with love, smile. Every time you smile, your heart chakra activates, and joyful love flows through your body. Keep smiling, allowing every cell in your body to smile, and notice what it feels like. You will probably feel your body bubbling with joy, so smile some more.
2. Now notice love building stronger and stronger in your cells until they overflow with love. As you feel every organ in your body overflowing and shining with love, smile again.
3. Allow your entire body to overflow and radiate love into your auric field, and beyond to bless life. Exhale love from your body, and on an inhale, breathe the great field of love back into your cells.
4. Keep radiating love out of your cells on the exhale and receiving love back into your cells on the inhale. Repeat this process until you feel the internal love vibration connecting to the external love vibration. Your body is a conduit to bridge your microcosm to the macrocosm.

Awareness 3: Your Sexual Energy Is Magnetized to Love

As we have talked about it in previous chapters, your sexual energy gets magnetized to love. Love spins your cells to create chakras. These spinning vortexes create a gravitational pull that calls the sexual energy to unite with them. Just like blood travels through your arteries and then into capillaries to nourish the cells, your sexual energy travels through your energy pathways to energize the cells. As soon as your sexual energy enters into your cells, a little explosion of energy takes place - sparking the cells with new life and consciousness. It is your sexual energy that helps bring the vibration of love into physical reality. Sexual energy is a very physical force, and it must be acted out. It is the sublimation of your sexual energy that turns love into a verb. This means that the dynamic experience of love can be created from talking, thinking, feeling, inspiring, guiding, explaining, kissing, touching, walking, dancing, and sleeping. Every time any part of you moves, you have the potential to generate love. The key is to become conscious of each awareness, that generates from each action. Love in physical motion brings many insights, and moments of enlightenment to the one who acts it out.

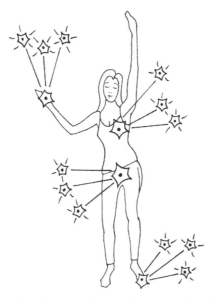

Figure 3: Your Sexual Energy Is Magnetised To Love

Movement Exercise - *refer to figure 3:*

1. Your sexual energy is a very intelligent force, and it knows exactly where to go and what to do. All it requires is for you to set it free and allow it to exist as a sacred force in your life. One of the easiest ways to awaken your sexual energy is to dance. Moving your arms, shimmying your hips, rotating your pelvis, and snaking your spine releases sexual energy and encourages it to travel through your body. As this occurs, you may feel joyful sensations popping, fizzing, and rippling inside as the sexual energy collides with the love in your cells. Every time you experience this, smile. Smiling deepens the experience, and it also helps you generate more love inside your body.
2. If you want to enhance the experience, gently touch the erogenous zones on your skin and allow your sexual energy to blossom in those areas. As you move, become more conscious of your sexual energy as it flows through your energy pathways - this will heighten your body's sensitivity.

3. Dancing for five minutes every day will help free your sexual energy to live as a sacred force inside of your body.

Awareness 4: The Heart

Once you honor your sexual energy as a sacred force, you can easily train it to unite your heart. When this occurs, a divine inner marriage takes place, and you become your own soul mate. Your sexual energy is always seeking union, and the greatest union you will ever have is with your heart. To be your own soul mate, changes forever, the way you relate to yourself and life. When you fulfill your heart with your sexual energy, the deep inner loneliness shifts, and your loving truth has the power to awaken. This teaches you that you can supply all the love you'll ever need all by yourself.

No longer will you need someone else to complete you; instead you fulfill yourself. You will, of course, desire to share life and intimacy with another person, but *sharing* is very different from *needing* and *demanding*. The overflow of self-love is what allows you to truly love someone else. When sexual energy finds a home in your heart, it will expand your heart chakra and fuel your loving truth to shine out into the world. Your sexual energy can then act as a bridge, connecting your entire being to the vibration of love that exists in life, and ultimately in the entire universe.

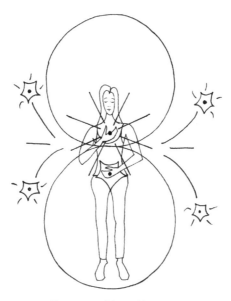

Figure 4: Your Heart

Movement Exercise - *refer to figure 4:*

1. To invite your sexual energy into your heart chakra, first place one hand on your heart and the other hand on your womb space or sexual palace. Visualize a figure eight moving between these two centers, helping them to unite.
2. Move your hips and rotate your pelvis to activate the sexual energy and allow it to freely move through your body. As this occurs, you may feel tremoring energy rippling up though your body. Make sure you smile every time you feel it collide with the love inside.
3. Using your breath and intention, direct your sexual energy up to your heart on the inhale, and on the exhale, breathe your sexual energy out of your heart chakra. Repeat this process until you feel your heart chakra bursting with love.
4. Eventually you can complete the energy circuit by inhaling sexual energy up to the heart and then exhaling the sexual energy through the heart chakra, directing it to unite with the sexual palace again. In this way you make love to yourself—a very beautiful and sensual experience.

Awareness 5: The Erogenous Zones

Your body is one big sexual palace, and every cell is designed to blossom with your sexual energy. We often limit our sexual palace to our genitals, but once your sexual energy moves toward the heavens, your entire body becomes a vessel of sensual delight. The ability for your sexual energy to blossom out of your cells, makes your inner beauty become your outer radiance. To have your sexual energy push your unique vibration of love out of every cell is the most wondrous sensation. It will warm your body with joy, bring a sense of contentment to your heart, allowing you to feel beautiful inside and out. To be able to blossom your unique vibration through your body at will, is a very empowering experience, one that will cure your need for approval. To achieve this, all you need to do is guide your sexual energy from the genitals to meet your erogenous zones. The erogenous zones store sexual energy throughout your body, and for most women they include the following areas: feet, inner thighs, hips, stomach, nipples, upper arms, neck, lips, mouth, ears, and head. Your erogenous zones are personal to you, and you may find other areas of your body that are easily stimulated. Eventually with practice your entire body can become one erogenous zone.

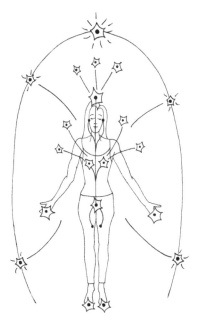

Figure 5: The Erogenous Zones

Movement Exercise- *refer to figure 5:*

1. Begin caressing your body. You might like to be naked for this exercise. Pay particular attention to your erogenous zones, and with a gentle touch awaken the sexual energy that exists there.
2. Every time you feel your sexual energy activating around your body, smile. Touch your lips and smile. Touch your ears, arms, breasts, and nipples, and smile. Touch your inner thighs and your sexual palace, and smile. Remember, smiling promotes love to flow, so as you awaken your body, feel your inner beauty shining through your skin.
3. When you inhale, contact your sexual energy in your sexual palace, and contract your muscles around it. Just like a pump, push your sexual energy up to your erogenous zones.

4. When you exhale, release your sexual energy through your erogenous zones and visualize your inner beauty becoming your outer radiance.

5. Practice doing this sequence to blossom other parts of your body. Direct your sexual energy to blossom through your arms, legs, head, eyes, and anywhere else you would like to feel your beauty shine.

Awareness 6: Kundalini

The awakening of Kundalini energy begins as soon as you step on to your spiritual path. The spiritual path, is the journey you take to become more conscious of the love that exists within and around you, so oneness can be experienced. The Kundalini energy can begin with pulsing sensations at the base of the spine, and then extend to electric surges that move through the spine and body. When this occurs, the central core of the body begins to open, and this allows the Kundalini energy to flow through and awaken the chakras. Cathartic experiences generate from every Kundalini awakening; whether from a small pulse to a massive surge, the Kundalini awakening energy is designed to break through old patterns stored inside the body. As it does, it charges and empowers the sexual energy, and encourages it to keep traveling up through the body. Kundalini energy seeks total liberation from the *maya*, a Sanskrit word that describes the material world as an illusion. Kundalini energy helps you transcend physical desire and illusion so you can truly experience love.

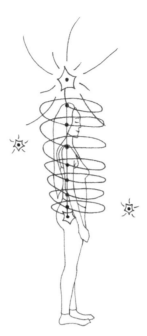

Figure 6: Kundalini

Movement Exercise - *refer to figure 6:*

1. The Kundalini energy is activated in different ways throughout your life, sometimes subtly and other times in more extreme ways. One of the best ways to maintain the health of your Kundalini energy is to do a simple chakra breathing exercise. To begin with, contact the Kundalini pulse at the base of the spine; this can be achieved by becoming more aware of it through intention or by moving the hips to activate the energy in the lower part of the spine.

2. When you locate the pulse of energy in the spine, breathe into it and allow it to become more active. As it does, you may feel energy shooting up your spine.

3. Inhale your awareness into the Kundalini energy at the base of your spine; exhale and allow the Kundalini to move up your body. Do this a few times.

4. On the next inhale, breathe the Kundalini up your spine to the first chakra, and then exhale the kundalini energy out through

the front of your first chakra and circulate it back to its origin at the base of the spine.

5. Repeat this process, stopping at each of the chakras all the way up to the crown. As you do this, your dormant sexual energy will start activating around your body. Make sure you smile when moments of love awaken in your cells!

Awareness 7: The Earth

Your body temple needs to be connected to the earth. It is important that you notice your body absorbing and being nourished by earth energy, on a daily basis. On a physical level, the fruit you eat and the essential oils that perfume your skin nourish your body. On an energetic level, the vibrations that the Earth itself emits nourish you. If you stand on the grass with bare feet, you might feel the subtle pulse of the earth coming up, through the soles, to feed your energy pathways. Most of us in the modern world are becoming more and more distracted and less connected to nature. Our bodies then slowly forget to invite the earth's energy in. But on your path of sensual enlightenment, you need the earth's energy to support the evolution of sexual energy through your body. Through awareness you can invite the earth's energy to keep rising through your body. As it does, you will notice it pushing your sexual energy to move upward as well. Just like a straw that drinks in juice, your energy pathways can drink the earth's energy all the way up to the top of your head. Your vagina also acts as a pump, and you can use the internal muscles of your sexual palace, to pull the earth energy into your womb space to support your sexual energy. As the earth's energy moves through the pathways of the vagina and sexual palace, the Kundalini energy at the base of the spine is stimulated to awaken. The earth is a vital ingredient in helping your sexual energy blossom and your energy connect to the heavens.

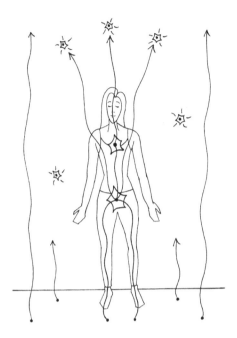

Figure 7: The Earth

Movement Exercise - *refer to figure 7:*

1. Stand outside on the grass and send your awareness down to your feet. Notice the earth's energy bubbling up from the ground and stimulating your feet.

2. Next visualize all your energy pathways extending from your feet, into the ground and drinking in the earth's energy. Feel the earth's energy rising up through your legs. Like a tree that wants to grow tall, the earth's energy will help to push your sexual energy up toward the heavens.

3. Notice the sensations that earth energy brings to your body, and the sensations it gives as it pushes your sexual energy upward. As this occurs you may feel yourself being nourished and supported from the inside out. Smile as the earth's energy, your sexual energy, and love collide inside of you.

4. Notice the orgasmic sensations of delight it creates inside your cells, and smile. Next, focus your awareness on your vagina, becoming aware of your intimate muscles. As you inhale, squeeze your vaginal muscles, and when you exhale, release your vaginal

muscles. Practice this a few times until you feel that your vagina is fully activated.

5. Next, inhale and contract your vaginal muscles, visualize your vagina drinking in the earth's energy. On the exhale, relax those muscles. Repeat this, allowing the earth's energy to fill your womb space and then move through your body.

6. If you would like to activate the Kundalini energy, you can also use your vagina muscles like a pump and direct the earth's energy to the base of the spine. As you do, allow the Kundalini energy to rise up your spine. This should be a very gentle and energizing experience.

Awareness 8: The Heavens

Your beautiful body temple needs nourishment from so many different forces. You are a multidimensional, multifaceted being that requires the sun, the stars, and the moon to nourish you. Just as you eat food with your mouth, every cell is able to open to receive nourishment from the cosmic forces. As plants derive nutrients from sunlight and exchange it into energy, your body does the same. The hunger we often feel as women is not because we need more food, but rather because we need more of the cosmos, more of our sexual energy, and more love. You are an energy being, and the cosmic forces will rejuvenate and supply your body with new information. Every star in the sky, is coded with a unique frequency of light, that can awaken your consciousness with new awareness. In particular, our closest star, the sun, is able to warm and charge our bodies like a battery. Moonlight is sunlight reflected and offers a softer "yin" form of nourishment. Through intention, you can call the different cosmic forces into your body, to feed your cells, and awaken you with heightened awareness. The ability for your body to transduce the heavens allows your energy body to expand into it. We can only become more, when we incorporate more into our lives. The energy of the heavens teaches us that there is an infinite amount of resources available to help support every need in our life's journey. Every star in the sky will awaken your body, mind, and soul when you remember how to relate to them.

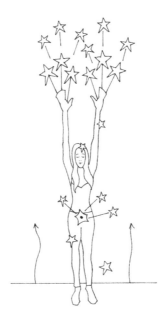

Figure 8: The Heavens

Movement Exercise - *refer to figure 8:*

1. Stand underneath a night sky and feel the immenseness of the stars above you. As you do this, you may notice your energy body expanding to connect with them. Higher and higher, you have the potential to stretch through the universe.

2. Feel the earth beneath your feet, and your sexual energy helping to push your aura into the heavens. For a moment let each star in the sky shine into you; see if you can feel the different frequencies.

3. Notice the feelings that dip and rise inside of you as each star kisses you. On an inhale, draw starlight into your body and witness each cell drinking in the illuminating light. On the exhale, let your cells reflect starlight back out to fortify your energy body.

4. Repeat this process until you glow with starlight. To heighten the experience, reach your hands up to the sky and guide starlight back to your body with your fingers.

5. On the inhale gather starlight, touch your erogenous zones with it, and smile. Then on the exhale, breath the starlight through

your body. Notice it tingling through your energy pathways to nourish your sexual energy.

6. You can repeat this process using sunlight, moonlight, planets, galaxies, or even by tuning into entire star constellations. The andromeda galaxy is my favorite.

Awareness 9: Cosmic Loving

As soon as your sacred sexual energy blossoms, it does two very beautiful things. Firstly, it helps to activate the divinity in everything it connects to. Secondly, it goes in search of the vibration of love that exists within the space of physical reality. In order for this to occur, you require lots of love and sexual energy to emit from your body. It is therefore important, that you keep cultivating your sacred sexual energy to be a powerful fuel. Every time you emit energy from your cells, you also create energy pathways that extend out and connect to life. Since your body can blossom in all different directions - from the front, behind and below, your energy pathways also extend out into all directions. This helps strengthen your auric field and energy body. It will also help you find the great field of love that exists all around you. Once your energy pathways are able to locate it, they can then begin to drink the high frequencies of love back into the body. It is the ability of the body, to open and receive, that gives you the exquisite sensation of being made love to by love itself. As this occurs, the body floods with so much love, that many ecstatic and orgasmic experiences take place. When the great field of love enters into each cell and chakra of the body, it can feel like a *lingam* entering a *yoni* (Sanskrit for a man's penis penetrating a woman's vagina). This will give the feeling of completion and expansion at the same time. The more you are able to receive love, the bigger and brighter your energy body becomes. This will give you the ability to go deeper into the great field of love, drawing even higher frequencies back into the body. The cycle continues, and is self-perpetuating, if you remain true to cultivating and awakening love in your body, mind, heart, and life.

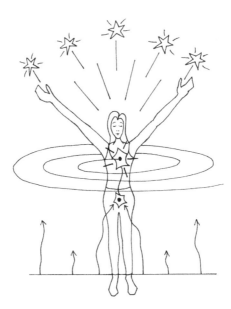

Figure 9: Cosmic Loving

Movement Exercise - *refer to figure 9:*

1.   1. Pull the earth energy up through your feet and into your sexual palace, letting your sexual energy ignite.
2.   Then on an exhale, send both the earth and sexual energy up to your heart. Allow them to blossom out of the heart chakra to bless your auric field.
3.   Raise your hands to the heavens, and on an inhale, call heaven's energy down through your fingers and into your heart chakra to unite with the love, sexual and earth energy that is there. On the exhale, breath all this energy out at once to bless your auric field.
4.   Continue this process until you feel your heart chakras expanding, and your auric field getting brighter and stronger. Allow your energy field to expand as it fills with more energy.
5.   Then on an exhale, open your auric field, and allow all of your beautiful energy to flow out and bless life.
6.   On the inhale, breath heaven, earth, love, and sexual energy into your heart. Exhale and breathe all of that amazing energy out into life.

7. Continue a few more times. Inhale and breathe heaven, earth, love, and sexual energy into your heart. Exhale and breathe all of that amazing energy out into life, except this time send it through the space between the molecules of reality to connect to the great field of love.
8. On an inhale, breathe the great field of love back into every cell of your body to nourish you. Exhale the orgasmic experience of love through your body, and smile.
9. Repeat this process until you feel the great field of love making love to your body. You may want to lie down for this.

Awareness 10: *Sensual Body Blossoming*

Sensually enlightened experiences are initiated by your ability to circulate sexual energy around your body, unite it to the love that exists in all of your cells, and then allow it to blossom through your skin. As you train your body to incorporate the heaven and earth energies as well, you will begin to feel your energy body growing to encompass more life. You will begin to feel more connected to the life around you. Trees, flowers, animals, and people will become more vibrant, and you will have a greater curiosity to connect to them from the space of love. It is in these moments that you can have a love affair with life. You can get intoxicated from the scent of perfumes, fall in love with trees, have a heart connection with an animal, or see the beauty in everyone that walks by. Every time love bursts from your being, you activate the divinity in the molecules that surround you to awaken as well. Through this act you help birth love into life, and you imprint every living thing with new information from which to evolve. You raise the consciousness of life around you from the vibrations you emit, and through this you awaken heaven on earth. The more your sexual energy is charged with love, earth and heaven's energies, the stronger it will become. All of these ingredients will empower your sexual energy to become stronger as a sacred force. From this heightened state, you will be able to use your sexual energy to manifest and magnetize to that which your heart desires. It will also become a source of power to increase your intuitive and psychic abilities, so you can heal and transform the lower vibrations of life around you. When your sexual energy allows your unique beauty to blossom, it gives you a presence that will light up every room you walk into. This presence is not just a glow—it is a field of energy that shifts the molecules in the room to come into alignment with love. Your presence also subtly projects your boundaries, so those around you can decipher what is appropriate behavior around and toward you.

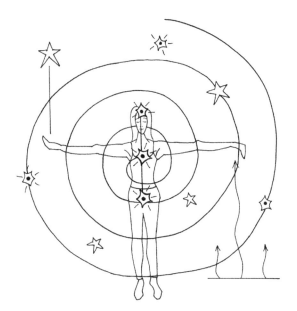

Figure 10: Sensual Body Blossoming

Movement Exercise - *refer to figure 10:*

1. Stand outside, naked if you dare, with your bare feet touching the earth and your head connecting to the heavens.
2. Stretch your hands out, one hand facing the heavens and one hand facing the earth, allow the energy of the earth and heavens to run through your hands and charge your heart to open with love.
3. Next, awaken your sexual energy by moving your body, guiding it to move upward with your hands, gently touching your skin and awakening all your erogenous zones to blossom with love and your sexual energy.
4. As you move, pull the earth's energy up through your energy pathways and vagina.
5. As you inhale, move the energy through your body, and as you exhale, feel the earth's energy blossoming though you.

6. Reach up to the heavens, and with your hands guide sun and starlight into your body.

7. On the inhale allow it to unite and charge all the energy inside of you, and on the exhale, let it release through your body.

8. Now try to do all of these actions at once. On an inhale, breathe both the heaven and earth energies into your body, letting them unite with the love and sexual energy that exists inside of you.

9. On an exhale, release all of the energy through every cell in your body until your auric field is nourished.

10. Repeat this again, building the energy on the inhale, and on the exhale releasing it through your cells and auric field and out to bless life. Continue this process, and if you like, you can practice directing your loving energy into trees, plants, flowers, or into the collective consciousness. Notice how fulfilling it is to give love back to life and allow more love to exist in reality.

Reflection:

1. After contemplating each awareness of sensual body blossoming and completing the movement exercises associated with it, reflect upon a) the body sensations each movement exercise gave to you; b) any insights or inspiring thoughts it gave to your awareness.
2. Which blossoming exercise was your favorite and most easy to do?
3. Which blossoming exercise did you find the most difficult? Why? What can you do to help master the exercise?
4. On a scale of one to ten (one being absent and ten being super vibrant), how would you describe your inner beauty as your outer radiance? Does it increase after doing the blossoming exercises?
5. What would your life be like if you could give yourself a score of ten? Who would you be? What would you do?
6. Can you think of any new ways to incorporate all the blossoming techniques of smiling, shining, sounding, moving, touching, and breathing?

7

Made of Starlight and Mud

*Y*our body is designed to open like a flower and emit love from the depths of your cells, through your body and out to bless life. It is the power of your sexual energy that helps blossom love through your body, and it is the combination of the love in your cells plus your sexual energy that releases everything that does not vibrate with love. This includes lower emotions such as guilt, shame, anger, and jealousy. Emotions are energy in motion; they are vibrations, and within them they hold memories and belief systems that form your perceptions and shape your reality. You are a vibrational being, and the love that lives within you is the highest and fastest frequency that exists, with the lowest being hatred. When you are clouded with lower emotions and thoughts such as sadness, guilt, shame, jealousy, and anger, they create waves of lower vibrations that clog and "muddy" the body. Conversely when you radiate emotions and thoughts that pertain to love, your physical body is rejuvenated, and the energy body expands with glowing and joyful presence.

'Your body expands with love and contracts with lower emotions.'

Your body expands with love and contracts with lower emotions. The lower emotions that clutter your body have come from negative beliefs, perceptions, hurts, defenses, confusion, self-doubt, karmic plus generational baggage, and collective consciousness drama, causing the energy in your body to contract. This contraction makes you feel deflated and disconnected from yourself. Your mud clogs the energy pathways and blocks your essence from flowing into your organs, and this can create disease or illness and inhibit your own connection to your heart. This then obstructs love flowing out to connect with others. The energy pathways in the body close, leaving you feeling caged in your body and trapped in your life. Your body temple then becomes a prison, inhibiting the freedom of your spirit to fully exist.

If your essence is restricted from connecting to life, you will be less able to manifest, because the screen of life is unable to locate you. Instead, all that gets presented are your troubles and your hurts, which then creates challenges in your relationships and obstacles in your life. You start to feel separate, isolated, and lost in a world where you don't belong. You may even wish you were someone else or feel so dense with lower emotions that you feel too disempowered to change. But this is all part of the process.

Your mud forms from your heart breaking and the love within descending and fracturing into lower emotions. The break usually occurs from an external event and gets created from an experience, another person, or your reaction to a situation. Every lower emotion that blocks your body is actually your inability to respond to an adverse situation with love. Your anger, hatred, jealousy, loneliness, and confusion are merely distorted reactions; often for various reasons you have also been programmed to respond in such a way.

Your "mud" is not bad; it is actually a very beautiful part of you. We are all born with "mud," and part of our journey is learning to evolve out of it. You may have referred to the "mud" as your shadow, your limited subconscious, those parts of you that are broken, lost, or confused, or the hidden, suppressed, or denied parts of you. All you need to do is learn to love the mud—loving those parts back to wholeness and newness. No part of you should ever feel rejected or unworthy; every part of you deserves to be loved. You are the only person in this entire universe that can love all of you. No one else can, and no one else will.

Like opening a flower petal by petal, you must learn to release your mud layer by layer, emotion by emotion, memory by memory, until you free yourself from the past and that which is not your authentic truth. The key to this process is to become aware that you have all the wisdom, intelligence, and guidance to be able to refine and evolve everything back to love. From this knowing you will begin your path of self-healing, not as a victim but as an empowered being who is free to transform everything. You just need to practice this until it becomes easy.

On this path you will learn to love every single part of you until it heals, evolves, and awakens. You will learn to forgive, get wiser in the truth of love, and become more careful with your actions and words so you minimize breaking love unnecessarily again. No longer can you project the damaged relationship you had with your mother, father, or some other past relationship onto the next person. No longer can you expect another person to heal the distortions inside you. As an evolved being, you must self-heal, and through the process learn to love your wounds and therefore love yourself even more.

'*Self- love teaches you how to self-heal.*'

It is through self-love that you learn how to self-heal. Self-healing will teach you about who you are, revealing your gifts and talents; it will bring much strength and empowerment because you have evolved out of your darkness. It is through self-healing that you discover yourself, that you get to know yourself. You become your own best friend, your own soul mate. When self-healing occurs, the love you have for yourself overflows to uplift others. All that you have evolved out of blesses all those around you with new teachings and a new awareness of love.

When you begin the journey to heal that which is out of alignment to your unique version of love, you indirectly become conscious of what was unconscious. To make the unknown known is a beautiful blossoming that ultimately brings you more awareness of who you are and the nature of the divine universe. It opens your intuition and aligns you to your authentic truth.

Your beautiful body is like a divine flower with millions of petals that long to awaken to the light of love. This movement of awakening the subconscious to become conscious is never-ending; it is a continuous unfolding. The path of enlightenment centers around this process and requires that everything in the subconscious evolves into the conscious so it can evolve into the superconscious. In other words, the contracted mud within you must be recognized so you can heal and return to love. The superconscious is the divine universe of love—this is your origin and your destination. As a woman, your sensual enlightenment comes from both returning and awakening your female body temple to become one with and reflect love.

Through this process of loving your "mud" and healing and discovering yourself, something very exquisite happens. Just as a light shone through a prism creates a rainbow, the lessons you learn from transforming your mud bring a very particular intelligence to you. This makes you a unique fractal of energy, because the light within you desires to blossom regardless of energetic obstacles. This allows the love within you to shine in a very unique way. Your "mud" is a blessing because it makes you a unique fractal of love.

'You are a unique fractal of love.'

To be a unique fractal of love means that you have evolved beyond your adversities and challenges by using the virtues, wisdom, integrity, and solutions that love brings. It means that you are mastering and creating your life through the power of love. Never before and never again will the great field of love have the opportunity to birth through the very unique position of your body temple. Your beautiful body and all the "mud" you carry within it is the perfect fertilizer for the purity of love to be able to transcend. The journey you take to awaken from broken love is completely unique; your journey toward enlightenment is essential to awaken the divine with new awareness. As you heal the broken love within, you not only restore heaven on earth, you participate in a divine evolution of expanding and making the absolute light more intelligent. Through this process love itself becomes wiser, more compassionate, and more courageous.

As you participate in the awakening of love through your body temple, you indirectly help the great field of love to evolve. Your evolution into love advances the teachings and the power of the great field of love, which then brings higher intelligence and more awareness to others so they, too, can evolve with more ease. In other words, the love that exists within you teaches the love that exists around you, and this is how you raise the consciousness of life to experience more love. You, beautiful woman, are both a unique fractal of love and a creator of love. Through your words, thoughts, actions, and feelings, you process that which is not love to become love. This makes you a generator of love as well. You hold the keys to unlock heaven.

The more you honor the path of love, the easier it will become to identify and heal the mud you were born into. The mud within gets created every time you experience love breaking. Your heart breaks when someone dear dies, when a relationship fails, when you miss out on an opportunity, or when someone betrays or shouts at you. The human body is ancient, and the broken love patterns inside of you are old, numerous, and complicated. Some are born from times of war, famine, poverty, and illness. Other patterns come from greed, abuse, betrayal, or the injustice of being unfairly treated. To master love means healing all of your corrupted definitions of love. This could include "love is painful," "love is abusive," "love always leaves," or "love always creates fights."

Corrupted Love Creates Mud

All corrupted love patterns accumulate over time and through the generations, stunting the path toward enlightenment. Generations upon generations of distorted love has been passed down from mother to daughter, father to son, father to daughter, and mother to son. As a result, many have been born into families where the love distortions have created abuse, jealousy, manipulation, aggression, rejection, abandonment, confusion, power plays, or just the simple inability to show affection and give love to each another. This creates twisted definitions of love where love equals pain or hurt, where love is jealous, mean, and possessive, or where love is cold, withholding, and without affection. Often one learns to substitute love with the lower vibrations of hate, manipulation, shame, guilt, and anger. When one is born into such a dynamic, the understanding of love is so corrupted that unfortunately one seeks out partners with the same patterns. On one hand like attracts like, and in familiarity there is a sense of safety. On the other hand, there is a desire to resolve the love conflict, and so one will subconsciously attract situations that are similar to their distortions in order to overcome them by reacting to them in a new way. But when relationships form from corrupted love, it takes a lot of awareness from both parties to resolve and evolve out of them. For some the mud can form an emotional poverty consciousness where there is never enough love or affection, or where love is the experience of abandonment and rejection. The reasons why someone might conclude that there is a lack of love are numerous. For example, this could be formed by being rejected by friends at school, being yelled at by one's parents, from having one's heart broken, experiencing grief, or feeling lonely or ashamed. Much of the internal struggles you experience are due to trying to solve the puzzles of broken love within so you can return to heaven.

When love breaks in your heart and your life, you feel as if *you* break. This feeling occurs because there are hundreds of energy pathways running between your cells, organs, and body parts. Every part of your body is just as intelligent as your brain and holds on to memories, trauma, and emotions that clog and entrap the body if they have not been processed by love. Broken love distorts the way energy flows through these energy pathways, creating illusions, illness, suffering, and grievances. Every time you experience love breaking, you break inside and fracture into multiple emotions such as hurt, loneliness, rejection, shame, guilt, anger, and confusion. This then makes your mud a very interesting collection of lower vibrations. Furthermore, if you corrupt love, you break the virtues of love, and this will disconnect you from your divine purpose of being blessed and blessing others. In these cases, the higher vibrations of heaven separate from the body's energy system. The body then contracts and forms an egoic identity that is selfish; it now has to survive in a "harsher, loveless world." This is a very barren reality, the love within and around feels very distant or completely absent. If often pulls one into believing that the material world is where you will find your happiness. In this separation, you will start buying your happiness instead of learning how to create it. Addictions to food, cigarettes, alcohol, drugs, shopping, codependent relationships, social media, and in extreme cases, self-harm, body image, and eating disorders can develop.

The mud that clogs your energy pathways forms out of two responses. The first comes from the external environment. This could be your mother yelling at you, your boss manipulating you, your partner cheating on you, or even your dog dying. Every action has a reaction, and the way you emotionally respond to a situation either liberates you or creates a block in the energy pathways. If you respond with compassion, wisdom, discernment, tolerance, or courage, you overcome the incident by applying love. This raises both your awareness and the situation to operate from a higher vibrational state and breaks the negative loop. If however, you respond in anger, jealousy, bitterness, fear, resentment, or guilt, you emit denser vibrations that create blocks and defenses in your energy body. Left unresolved, this will inhibit your ability to both receive and give love. In turn, it will make situations and relationships more complicated because you'll begin to operate from your mud as opposed to the love that lives deeper inside you. When this occurs, you can find yourself overreacting or being defensive, judgmental, or anxious. Over time the mud within builds until you begin feeling imprisoned in your body and trapped in your life. Your mud locks you in the past and inhibits your energy from being present and creating a brighter future.

Conflicts arise when the love deep within your cells tries to shine out but hits the mud built in your energy pathways. Two things can happen: either you will accept this deflated state as normal and gradually disconnect from the love that rings through your cells, or you will choose to transform your mud through self-healing so you can evolve out of it. It is by choosing the latter that begins the journey into self-love. Having deep compassion for your own suffering means that you allow the healing properties of love to emit from your cells into your mud and transform it. By loving all your inadequacies and lower emotions, you will also indirectly learn how to love other people's shortcomings. This will help them to become compassionate with themselves so they, too, can evolve into love.

'The better you are at generating self-love, the
more compassion you will have for life.'

It is only through this sometimes very painful journey of recovering from corrupted love that you become stronger at generating self-love. You have more compassion for life because you have learned to forgive. You become wiser in love and more careful with your actions and words so that you minimize breaking love unnecessarily again. You recognize how precious, delicate, and refined love is. As you untangle and transform your lower self, you free your energy pathways to flow with the energy of love again, and you free your spirit to experience love in your life. This is the true freedom you seek.

The more aware of your body you become, the more it will reveal its intelligence to you. Your body is a most amazing compass, and it will reveal illness or disorder when you are out of alignment with love. This is how your body becomes your own guru. When you are on the right path, you will feel joy, rushes of energy, and inspiring thoughts that pull you forward. When you vibrate with the virtues of love regularly, you feel more alive, and you have the fuel you need to enjoy more life more often. As you feel the love sparkling inside of you, you can say yes to new projects, ideas, inspirations, and creations. The clearer you feel in your body, the freer you will feel in life. This expansion grants the space needed for more love to emit from your cells in your aura. This then magnetizes more of your sexual energy to move through your body, which creates a stronger life force, making it easier to transmit your soul urges onto the screen of life so you can create changes in your reality.

Brocken Love in the Female Body

A woman's body has an extraordinary capacity to experience and generate love. Her path to enlightenment depends on her ability to embody love. It is love that strengthens a woman's psyche to be wise; it is love that empowers her heart to be courageous; it is love that awakens her body to be ecstatic; and it is love that supports her soul to live in freedom. A woman will never be happy unless she lives from and within love. It is only from this stance that she will be able to live in all her magnificence and truly be able to express her divine power. Just as broken love has passed through your family generation by generation, broken love has also passed through the female psyche generation by generation for centuries upon centuries. Many atrocities have been experienced that have caused the female heart to collapse, her intuition to be lost, and her sexual energy to be shamed into nonexistence. Such events include sexual slavery, the burning of witches and with it their right to heal, the denial of goddess and nature worship, arranged marriages, or living in patriarchal societies where women have been silenced from making important decisions about law, education, health, politics, and economics. Every woman that has been broken before you may vibrate inside of you asking to be healed. It could be the wounds of your mother, her mother, the women of your culture, your religion, or women that were suppressed by the rules of your country or political system. These women may ring inside of you and ask that you heal the broken female psyche of humanity. Although many today are pushing past the obstacles of their female past, you may still need to liberate yourself from the following illusions:

- The corruption experienced by your mother and all the women down your matriarchal or female genetic line. This could include inherited female reproductive and hormonal disorders, depression, domestic violence/abuse, or the enslavement to the house, children, and husband.
- The emotional wounds created by a mother who is jealous, absent, aggressive, manipulative, mean, or is unable to communicate love. Plus, the negative impact it has on one's relationship to self and other women.
- The historical atrocities women have experienced throughout history such as sexual slavery, rape, or religious and cultural persecution.
- The laws and social rules enforced from a patriarch-dominated society that may hinder your ability to become a powerful woman.
- The exclusion of women being able to own property, have their own businesses, and generate an income, which inhibits your ability to step into your own abundance.
- The exclusion of being able to make changes in political, economic, and educational systems.
- The impact of beauty becoming a commodity whereby women have been taught to buy their beauty instead of becoming it.
- The warped perception of femininity and sexuality that comes from the collective consciousness, particularly from pornography and the media.
- The denial of sexual energy being a source of vitality or the concept that it is a sin.
- The stories of female identity that have been passed down through fairy tales, keeping a woman weak in a vulnerable identity.
- The illusion that finding a soul mate will complete you and that you will live happily ever after.

These wounds ring deep through the female collective consciousness and may cause you to become overly responsible, leak your power, and disconnect your body from the innate gifts that are coded within. Such corruptions have resulted in many health issues, including reproductive disorders, menstruation issues, hormonal imbalances, thyroid disorders, infertility, birth traumas, anxiety, and depression. When love breaks so deeply, it creates so many low emotions that the mud clogging the energy pathways eventually manifests as disease in the physical body. To be disconnected from the magic of your female body is devastating. For some, body image issues and eating disorders develop, while others experience addiction, jealousy, and comparison. Some may even go a little crazy when they feel too broken to generate love.

When the female heart breaks, her whole body breaks, and when love is not generated, the sexual energy within is unable to find what it would otherwise be magnetized to. When sexual energy is lost and disconnected from the heart, anxiety can surface, spinning a woman into self-doubt, confusion, and depression. This often causes her to seek "love" outside of herself, which can lead to much disappointment. When a woman operates from a broken heart, she is needy and demanding. Her desperation can lower her standards and compromise her truth, further breaking her heart and lowering her self-esteem. A downward spiral into unworthiness then develops. The key to lasting happiness is to generate self-love first, so it can overflow from you to lift another in love. To expect someone else to complete you is an illusion that the female psyche often gets lost in.

When a woman's heart breaks, her sense of oneness with herself and the connection she has to the great field of love breaks as well. Her head feels separate from her heart, and her sexual energy will lose its ability to sublimate through the body. Before my sexual energy learned to sublimate from my base to my crown chakra, I often felt like I split into three different people. My mind took over as being hardworking, practical, judgmental of both myself and others, obsessed about achieving, and neurotic about my weight and how to achieve a better body shape. My mind overpowered my heart, which learned to deny my desires and collapsed into a feeling that I "was wrong" and "not good enough." My sexual energy had an untamed force of its own and would override the confusion in my heart and demands of my head. It would lead me to relationships both good and bad and often got me attracted to situations that damaged my growth. Then my head would go into self-blame, my heart would go into shame, and my sexual energy that wanted another adventure got excited to find more trouble. It was a cycle of self-destruction.

This is because the energy pathways that would have otherwise coalesced through the heart center became clogged with lower emotions, and this created a further disconnect. From this position, the mind, heart, and sexual energy become three separate beings, often pulling one in three separate directions if they are not united with love.

When your head disconnects from your heart, you experience an increase in negative and critical thinking because your thought processes are no longer filtered with love. When the sexual energy is unable to reach the head, your thoughts become foggy, your intuition weak, self-doubt increases, and reality is perceived as more problematic. When your mind and sexual energy are unable to anchor in your heart, your heart energy becomes weak, and instead of being able to shine out with joy into life, it collapses into lower emotions. This is true for each of your chakras; if they are not supported by love, intelligence, and sexual energy, they will collapse inwards and keep you locked in a lower vibrational consciousness like a broken record. When your heart is broken, the love that emits from your body diminishes and your sexual energy has no will to ascend; making it impossible for you to complete your journey to sensual enlightenment. This is a tragic place for any woman to be in. Heartbreak can debilitate some women for years—some for a whole lifetime.

'Your heart is so powerful and yet so vulnerable at the same time.'

Your heart is so powerful and yet so vulnerable at the same time. Every heartbreak you have experienced is an opportunity for you to awaken into a greater understanding of love. Each heartbreak can give you wisdom and discernment. Every heartbreak you recover from will empower you to stand stronger, act bolder, and speak louder. Each one will teach you how to be authentic and have empowered boundaries so you ensure greater respect and love from others. Every heartbreak will teach you how to love yourself and all your adversities until you heal every part of your body and every aspect of your life. Each heartbreak will make you stronger so that you cannot be broken again. As you master the path of love, you will master the ability to transform any broken heart or corrupted love experience with greater ease and more efficiency.

Human life will always present experiences that will break your heart, but over time through the experience of transcending them, you will master being present with all the dynamic qualities of love. Every heartbreak you heal from will require you to incorporate a virtue of love, wisdom, wonder, courage, passion, love, freedom, generosity, compassion, desire, dignity, faith, or the implementation of harmony. Some heartbreaks will teach you how to master one virtue of love; others will require that you implement many to transcend. For example, you may not have gotten the job you wanted. You may have felt rejected, disappointed, and heartbroken that your life has failed. But the simple virtue of faith reminds you that something more perfect is available. Faith will wash away the disappointment and strengthen you with the energy to keep looking for another job. Or maybe you have been in a long-term relationship that has caused many heartbreaks over the years. Maybe there have been arguments, infidelity, addictions, financial issues, or an incompatibility of your core values. Eventually you come to a point where the relationship needs to end. Such a choice would make you call upon many virtues so transformation can take place. Maybe you call upon the virtues of freedom and wonder, so a more aligned life can become available to you, the virtue of courage to confront your partner and end the relationship, the virtue of compassion to help yourself heal and move on, and then allow new desires to create new life.

Through the journey of recovering from heartbreak, you will birth yourself as a unique fractal of love. Every heartbreak is a blessing in disguise—all you have to do is master your ability to transcend through it. Remember that you are love, you come from love, you are surrounded by love, and love exists within every cell of your body.

As you heal your heart, you will also help your body to release the mud that clogs your energy pathways so they can flow with love again. When love flows, your sexual energy finds its purpose to ascend and sublimate through the body. Your sexual energy fuels the love within you to radiate out into your auric field so you can bless life. The more love you are able to project, the more empowered you will feel about your identity, the healthier your relationships are, and the more helpful you are to your community. You become more aware of your environment, more connected to the cosmic universe, and you become aware of the subtle and unseen worlds of angels, fairies, and tree and animal spirits. As I became more aware, I would often walk past trees and feel them energetically cleansing my aura, or they would call me to stand at their roots, with my spine against the trunk so my energy field could straighten and grow taller. Other times an animal would cross my path, and every time my being extended love toward it, I could feel the animal passing on a message. Squirrels would scuttle by, telling me to slow down, and birds would show me how to have greater vision for my life.

Releasing your mud is a lifelong but very beautiful process once you get through the dense layers at the beginning. Enlightenment is a never-ending journey. The more you awaken, the more you realize how much more awakening is ahead of you. This pulls the next layer of mud to the surface to transform. It's a process of continuous blossoming, one that will never end. Love is an infinite force; as soon as you awaken to it, you realize there is more to awaken to. And so the journey into love continues indefinitely.

Reflection:

1. Which lower emotions do you experience the most?
2. Which high vibrational emotions do you experience the most?
3. Explore your timeline and reflect upon all the heartbreaks you have experienced. What were your biggest lessons?
4. Where does your "mud" come from—family, experiences, society?
5. How does your "mud" affect the vibrancy in your body?
6. Do you suffer with any female health issues, such as hormone imbalance, thyroid problems, or pregnancy issues?
7. Explore the distorted female consciousness or beliefs that you may still carry from your culture, religion, or ancestry. Describe.
8. What does it mean to be a unique fractal of love?
9. What makes you a unique fractal of love?
10. What lessons and wisdoms of love do you give to the world?

8

The Lotus Transcends from Her Mud

Just as a lotus flower transcends from the mud to become a beautiful flower, you too must awaken out of your "mud" so you can operate from the truth of your existence. Evolving out of your lower emotions turns your mud into a rich soil. Your mud is a very beautiful part of you, and the lessons you learn from it will bless you with many abilities that aid your evolution into love.

Untangling Your Emotions

You must learn to feel comfortable with every emotion, from anger to sadness to jealousy to joy. Every emotion you have is valid and should never be censored, diluted, denied, or repressed. Every emotion that exists within you has a story locked within it—these are your memories, your past experience, your history, thoughts, judgments, illusions—and as you unravel your emotions, you free your energy to become you. And "you" are a very unique vibration and energy signature in this universe. You do not need to be clouded by that which is not you.

Your emotions help you navigate through life, and the more you transcend your lower, emotions, the more stable you will feel inside. This will indirectly help your psychic abilities increase. Every lower emotion that lives within you distorts the way you see the truth. The more you are able to vibrate with love, the clearer you will be able to see the spectrum of reality going on within and around you.

'By transcending your lower emotions, you discover your authentic truth.'

Every lower emotion you experience is merely a collapsed virtue of love. For example, sadness is the collapsed virtue of ecstasy; unworthiness forms when one's desires cannot be materialized; judgments form when there is a lack of compassion; and doubt exists when there is no faith. The aim of the game is to sit with each lower emotion and learn to untangle it until every part of you returns to love. As you guide yourself back to love, you will also learn the tools to help guide others back to love. Through the process of returning your shadows to love, you raise your vibration and emit more light into this world.

I suffered with anxiety and an eating disorder between the ages of ten and twenty-four. This caught me in a turmoil of self-hatred, self-rejection, and severe criticism. My journey of recovery was not about finding the perfect diet or becoming the perfect body shape. It was about acceptance. I had to learn to appreciate the parts of my body that I hated, and I had to make peace with myself so my internal battle and all the negative thinking could end. The cycle of my eating disorder resolved only when I learned to have complete compassion with all of who I was. Especially the "fat" and "ugly" parts. This process of self-love also helped me to become a better intuitive healer because I learned to go into the depths of human suffering and transform it in a very caring and nurturing way.

Every lower emotion you transcend will teach you something very valuable about your past, your present, and your future. Through this journey of transcending the lower parts within you, you will discover your authentic truth. To know who you are inside out will increase your sense of self-worth, which makes you feel empowered to be a unique individual who is unafraid to express it.

By mastering this technique, you increase your emotional intelligence, and this improves your ability to discern the emotional truth of others. This is extremely valuable because it teaches you how to decipher the true intentions and motivations behind another person's actions. From here you will indirectly develop your intuitive depth, which is the ability to see through people by understanding their truth, their inadequacies and where they are out of alignment in their life. This helpful skill will teach you how to deal appropriately with others. Sometimes you may need to avoid someone because they are operating out of alignment, and other times you will have deep compassion, understanding, and trust for another because you can sense their truth. You may already do this to some degree, and in advance cases you may receive extra psychic awareness such as premonitions, flashes and guidance that reveal more of the other person's "story."

As I learned to love myself and all of my hurts, shadows, shyness, unworthiness, anxiety, confusion, self-doubt, the experiences that created them, the dark memories that made them resurface, and the corrupted judgments that formed because of them, something very beautiful happened. The distortions that were jaded evolved out of being corruptions into an inner force of love which stabilized me into feeling peaceful. This peace brought emotional stillness, which in turn quieted my mind until I could sense the wisdom of the universe guiding me to understand the truth of reality. Instead of feeling conflicting emotions every time I interacted with life and people, I felt a deep wisdom informing me when to make connections and when to avoid them. This kind of energy also encouraged me to eat certain foods, listen to certain music, or go to certain places. Often the love inside would turn into a sense of power when I had to make certain decisions or confront people. It would flash around my clients, showing me the colors in their auras, their spirit guides, or their talents which they needed to remember. The clearer I became, the clearer I could experience the love with and around those communicating with me.

Below is a list of lower emotions and how you can return them to love. You may feel that you resonate with certain emotions more than others. The key is to train your awareness to find the path that leads from the

113

lower emotion back to the virtue of love. At the end of this chapter, there is a practical outline for achieving this.

How to Return Your Emotions to Love

1. Sadness/Loneliness Returns to the Ecstasy of Love

You experience sadness and loneliness every time you sense that you have been rejected or abandoned by someone. It could be from not having friends at school, being teased, or growing up in a family that didn't express affection. Sadness is the emotion felt from rejection, which then creates loneliness. Loneliness is the feeling that is created when you feel separate from everything. This deeply isolating place creates depression—and even suicide in extreme cases. These emotions can present as an energy within that retracts from life. The only way out of the depths of separation is by not expecting anyone to provide you with love. Instead, you must remember that you come from love, and through that simple acknowledgment, you will begin to become aware that the infinite pool of love within you is capable of filling your sadness and loneliness. When you work with sadness and loneliness in a conscious way, you may feel a cleansing as the grief passes through you; then there is rejuvenation and a rebirth into a new sense of self. The ecstatic pulses of love that live in every cell of your body breathe life back into you so you can celebrate yourself as alive, and this will relieve any sense of separation that you may have. From here sadness returns to happiness, and loneliness to the joy of being reconnected to love. The ecstasy of love returns when you choose to fill yourself with the love that exists within. Through this process you will learn to become responsible for the joy in your own life. Take yourself out on a date, join a group where you can socialize, or paint until you feel you've expressed your soul. Eventually this joy will connect you back to life and others again.

2. Confusion/Anxiety/Uncertainty Return to Wonder

Confusion and anxiety usually occur from an experience you could not make sense of. Perhaps you were lied to or given the wrong information, or maybe you grew up in an environment that was unstable and unpredictable. Confusion develops when there is not enough information to help you solve a challenge. Anxiety occurs when you try to solve the puzzle with the wrong solutions. Uncertainty forms when your solutions don't work, and you feel at the mercy of another person's decision. All of these emotions can create the energetic pattern of panic or falling through quicksand with no way out. Healing these emotions requires you to stop. Stop looking for a solution; stop trying to find a way out; stop listening to the thousands of thoughts running through your mind. It is only when you find the quiet within that the sense of inner wonder can emerge. Wonder is the ability to trust in an abundant universe that is always working in your favor. Often in ways that you can't even imagine. To move out of confusion, you must let go of the belief that your limited ability can solve the problem. Instead you must move into the knowing that love supplies an infinite amount of solutions. From this place of awe, anxiety can be replaced with gratitude, and uncertainty can return to trust. When we move out of theses chaotic emotions, we remember that we can feel inspired by love.

3. *Restriction/Imprisonment Returns to the Freedom of Love*

Certain emotions make you feel trapped, as though you have no choice or ability to change a situation. Restriction implies that there are rules, laws, and obligations that have been imposed upon you and go against your truth. This could include cultural values, religious views, family traditions, or socially acceptable behavior. Sometimes these are imposed through another's manipulation, force, or control. Other times, it is because you believe that you have to comply in order to maintain peace and harmony. Imprisonment occurs when those restrictions have forced you into compliance and you can no longer discern your own truth. You begin to feel trapped—in service to others and not to your higher truth. This will then make you feel as if you have no choice but to comply. Emotions of restriction and imprisonment create a sense of being bound to a certain paradigm. But through the freedom of love, you become aware that you always have a choice and you are not obligated to follow another person's rules. Freedom teaches you that nothing can ultimately control or suppress you. It is a transformative energy, and its sole purpose is to liberate you from that which does not come from love. The journey into freedom may mean that you remove yourself from certain people, take a break from traditions, and move out of feeling guilty for not fulfilling certain obligations. As you cut the ties, you free your spirit to live your life, not someone else's.

4. *Unworthiness/Failure/Apathy Returns to the Desire of Love*

The emotions of unworthiness, failure, and apathy are akin to feeling only half alive. There is a sense of pointlessness to life, often accompanied by listless feelings and depression. Unworthiness surfaces when you get excited about your truth followed by a sabotaging feeling that says you are not good enough to have it. Unworthiness often occurs as a result of your own critical thinking, or when the critical thinking of family members or partners belittles and diminishes your sense of self. This can then translate into "bad luck" or feeling that things never work out for you. When doors keep closing on your desires, exhaustion follows, which then turns into failure. If this continues the willingness to live new life fades and all desires die, resulting in apathy.

However, this very barren place can be a blessing in disguise. When doors and opportunities do not open in your life, it is a reminder that you are out of alignment with your true path. Apathy energetically looks listless with no active life force; unworthiness looks like self-rejection in which one continuously sabotages their light, and failure presents as a boulder of disappointments that squash the life force. However, within apathy and unworthiness there is a stillness, and if you center yourself in that stillness, you will be able to let go and detach from all that you have been identifying with or striving for. The exhaustion will go, the sense of failure will go, and so will the apathy and unworthiness. This place of stillness requires letting the old die completely so that the new can rebirth. When this occurs, new desires will spark inside of you, and you will relate to yourself in a whole new way. The slate must be wiped cleaned in order to reset your desires and live a full life again. Ask yourself, "What parts of me need to die in order for my desires to exist again?"

5. *Selfishness/Greed Return to the Exchange of Love*

Selfishness and greed both stem from the inability to share and exchange love. This usually develops from the absence of love in childhood, where one has experienced love from lack instead of abundance. This can happen when parents abandon, ignore or forget you. Perhaps parents considered their work more important than you, or perhaps you grew up in a family with drug and alcohol addiction, or with parents who lacked empathy and the ability to communicate affection. Selfishness comes from the fear that if you share, you will not receive back anything in exchange. Instead you become possessive of the little you have, and this behavior eventually leads to greed, which is an obsession with receiving versus giving. Selfishness and greed have an energetic pattern that resembles a black hole, where everything gets pulled into the deep void of lack in the body. The only way out of this paradigm is remembering that love is abundant and that in order to receive, you must also learn to also give. It is through giving that you will learn to receive as a blessing, not as a possession. From this space you will then learn that giving brings more pleasure than receiving, and you will develop an overwhelming desire to share with others. This motion ushers a sense of community where you feel motivated to support charities or causes that benefit the greater good. This is the exchange of love, where kindness bequeaths kindness.

6. *Jealousy/Manipulation Returns to the Generosity of Love*

Jealousy and manipulation come from being denied, rejected, or displaced from love and becoming upset when someone else gets to experience it. Jealousy is an envious resentment that secretly wants to take the joy from another in order to satisfy the self. Sometimes you might be jealous of another person's success, their partner, their clothes, or their looks. Energetically jealousy extends from the body as a dark, gooey energy that projects onto another to diminish their shine. The real reality is that your jealousy actually diminishes your shine and will hold you back from blossoming into your unique self. Every jealous thought highlights that you are capable of achieving that which you are jealous of. It can also reveal that you have dormant talents you are underutilizing. For example, being jealous of someone wearing designer clothes can be a sign for you to get more creative with the wardrobe you have. Being jealous of someone being more beautiful than you is a sign for you to adore and love yourself more. The key is to turn jealousy into motivation.

Manipulation is actively undermining someone or persuading them to give you what you desire without honoring their truth. Energetically manipulation is wrapping your energy around another person as a way to coerce, control, or delude them. It often manifests in the form of energetic hooks that can imprison another into compliance. Most manipulations stem from jealousy; the difference is that those who are jealous keep it hidden as an internal feeling, whereas those who use manipulation act upon their jealousy in greedy ways. Both of these emotions stem from a great sense of lack, and the only way to overcome them is to be extremely generous with yourself. You must love yourself more than you need someone else to love you. You must supply yourself with everything you would otherwise coerce and extract from another. You choose to gift yourself with the skills and items you have been jealous to possess. This process will teach you that you can raise yourself to the next level, and a sense of pride and fulfilment will replace the twisted emotions of lack. One of the hardest lessons to master is the ability to love yourself more than anyone else can.

7. *Judgment/Comparison Returns to Compassion:*

Judgment and comparison are emotional reactions created when you stay locked in your limited paradigm and cannot see beyond your own imposed rules and regulations. Many of your judgments have been subconsciously formed through the generations and from the collective consciousness, which can include perceptions about other races, religions, and social status. Judgment creates a barrier between you and others, stopping you from seeing the truth of love that exists within them. Comparison forms from a judgment of another person which you then apply to yourself. You might judge someone for being beautiful, and then judge yourself for not being beautiful enough. Both judgment and comparison block the flow of love between you and others, as well to yourself. They slowly replace feeling connected to feeling isolated. It is only through compassion that one learns to no longer discriminate. Compassion melts away the labels and perceptions that separate, teaching you to accept the differences. Through this process you will recognize that everything in this universe is unique, and you will begin to understand the infinite amount of ways that love can express itself.

8. *Ignorance/Blame Returns to the Wisdom of Love*

Ignorance and blame are opposites, but both of these emotions stem from the inability to express the wisdom of love. Ignorance comes from your inability to comprehend the truth of a situation. Sometimes it's due to a lack of knowledge, while at other times it's because it is easier to play dumb and unaware. Blame, on the other hand, completely skips the idea that there may be another side to the story and issues an aggressive judgment instead. When one blames another person, they choose not to take responsibility for their role in the situation. Ignorance often brings an energetic pattern of a void or avoidance, whereas blaming projects the negative energy from the inside out. Both ignorance and blame forget that there is always a deeper awareness that can be accessed to bring resolution. In every moment, in every situation, challenge, and obstacle, you have access to the wisdom of love. This is the ability to awaken to a higher solution or understanding that brings resolution to a problem. The wisdom of love teaches that there is greater awareness beyond your own thoughts.

9. *Dishonesty/Shame/Guilt Returns to the Dignity of Love*

Dishonesty, shame, and guilt form every time the integrity of love has been abused. Guilt emerges when you know you have betrayed love. This could be from lying, cheating, or manipulating someone out of a selfish desire. Shame occurs when you have been the victim of another's dishonesty. It usually occurs if you have been abused and the humiliation makes you want to keep the trauma a hidden secret. The energy of shame can feel like a heavy cloak, whereas the energy of guilt can twist you in knots. Both these emotions lock you in the past where you often relieve the scenario out in your mind again and again. When someone is dishonest, they break the virtues of love from existing in their life. This can be very painful because there is a knowing that they have inflicted this divine separation upon themselves and someone else. However, every wrong action teaches us many valuable things about right action. This teaches the one who feels guilty that there is a need to forgive their misdeeds and correct their future actions. The one who feels shame learns that they do not have to be branded by another person's actions. These emotions remind us that beneath our disturbances, our ethical backbone always exists, and so the integrity of love returns us to live a noble life again.

10. *Fear/Coward Returns to the Courage of Love*

Fear and cowardliness come from the inability to change a situation. Fear is created by absolute powerlessness compounded with terror of not surviving. It is the inconsolable panic that arises from fear that paralyzes one into feeling completely disempowered to make a change. Cowardliness is different; one is aware they have the power to change the situation, but is afraid to actually act upon it. When one acts cowardly, one often experiences deep regret afterward. Fear can often present as the energy within collapsing in disempowerment, and cowardliness can present as an energetic pattern of being too weak to progress. Both fear and cowardliness need to call upon the courage of love to help them transcend their challenges. Courage offers confidence and a boldness because it remembers that there is a force greater than the self that can be called upon at any time. When this is remembered, one can step out of their fear and be motivated to make a change.

11. *Mistrust/Suspicion/Doubt Returns to the Faith of Love*

Mistrust, suspicion, and doubt are emotions that form when you are unable to trust a situation or a person. Energetically they present as a paranoid energy that can't locate the love existing within or beyond you. Suspicion and mistrust usually develop if you have been deceived in the past. On one hand, it is good to be weary of anyone who is out of alignment. On the other, it can create a false reality where you avoid all interactions for the fear of being used or taken advantage of. Then when the illusion breaks, you are left feeling uncertain about what the real truth is and who you can rely on. Doubt develops when your sense of trust gets broken time and time again. Usually it occurs when one views situations like a child, where everyone is seen as being more knowledgeable than you. Doubt, suspicion, and mistrust occur when one forgets that there is a greater guidance available to rely upon. These emotions ask you to look beyond the reality in which you live, and send your awareness into the love that surrounds you to get the answers you seek. It asks you to step beyond your own paradigm, as well as others' paradigms. The faith of love teaches you that in every moment you have access to a higher intelligence that will guide you to the truth.

12. *Drama/Disruption Returns to the Harmony of Love*

Drama and disruption as emotions can be extremely destructive if left unchecked, but they can also be the instigators that break down old paradigms that no longer serve you. Drama occurs when you cannot transcend your lower emotions and project them onto other people and situations. Disruptions are usually formed from external events that change your life completely. It could be from someone dying, moving into a new home, or changing jobs. All disruptions require you to readjust to your new paradigm and in doing so require you to release old habits and patterns so new ones can form. The chaos comes when you do not release the old and try to reapply old patterns to the new situation. You will find yourself quickly out of alignment and battling with the new circumstances. Drama, chaos, and disruption all require you to surrender to change and transcend your lower emotions and patterns before they create more disturbances. The lesson is allowing the change to reconfigure your life to a greater experience of love. Only then will you recognize that every situation, and every person, is there to help you create harmony so, love can exist as a stable force in your life.

13. *Hatred/Anger and Resentment Returns to the Creation of Love*

Hatred, anger, and resentment are the lowest and most dense emotions because they stop love from existing. When anger arises, it's usually because you are perceiving or experiencing injustice. Injustice occurs any time you feel unfairly treated through rejection, betrayal, mistreatment, or violation on a physical, emotional, or spiritual level. Anger often arises when you feel threatened and you feel the need to protect your space. Sometimes you do need to express your anger and your boundaries, but in ways that do not hurt people and ruin relationships. Often anger can overtake your ability to be rational because it stimulates the adrenals to move into fight mode. But since you have the ability to communicate, you must allow the intelligence in your anger to speak, not your aggression. Your anger will then turn into power.

Resentments are suppressed anger that builds over a period of time.

There can be so many layers of resentment that you no longer have any awareness as to why you feel so indignant. Grumpy old men are the perfect example. Resentment, like anger, creates a very hard energy in the body, and if left to fester, it can create a bitterness that rejects all love and joy from existing in a person's life. The agony of being betrayed or mistreated is so painful that barriers of resentment are put up to protect the individual from more hurt. Hatred occurs when resentment becomes so intense that any sense of love or self-love gets squeezed out of existence. The bitterness might become so extreme that love is no longer generated or accepted by the individual. Hatred, anger, and resentment all lock us in the past and can often leave us feeling vengeful.

In order to transcend hatred, anger, and resentment, you must remember that you have the power to transform every situation. You are not subject to circumstances, nor do you need to fester about being a victim or begrudge the past. Once you acknowledge that you can call upon love as a creative force that transcends the situation, forgiveness immediately arises to release you from the past, and a flood of insights is granted that causes your thinking to evolve. This frees you to stand strong in the awareness that you are the creator of your own destiny. From this space, the blame, the pain, and the memories can be liberated. As soon as this occurs, you let go of the torture created by the past and actively choose to generate new life. The creation of love allows the old to die so the new can be rebirthed. It is also an act of forgiveness as you are freed to create new beginnings.

The Five Keys to Unlocking Your Mud

Unlocking your mud can be a simple, drama-free process. It merely requires you to move through five easy steps. At first it may be a little difficult because the love within you is trying to blossom through your denser layers. This may make you feel stuck, uncertain, or confused as to why a particular bit of mud has formed. This is all normal—just relax, be patient, and hold yourself in a space of compassion until the mud melts and you can feel the love within you shining. Remember, beneath all that mud lives the ecstatic vibration of love. Set an intention to keep connecting to it, and the intelligence of your body will do the rest. Although the process below is ordered from one to five, there is no ultimate order, and you may find a different step is more appropriate to focus on first.

1. *Recognize Your Mud.*

The blocked energy inside your body is ultimately made up of layers of emotions that have been broken or fragmented away from love. As a woman, you have been designed to feel deeply, but often you have not been taught how to process and befriend the overwhelming emotions that leave you feeling uncertain, confused, and disorientated. Women by nature tend to hold on to emotions, which means that they are loaded with many layers of unexpressed feelings. For some, there are so many layers that numbness develops because there is too much to process. Numbness merely needs a lot of self-love until it feels safe to feel again.

Close your eyes and allow yourself to become aware of your body, then wait to feel the first layer of mud to surface. You may feel it as a block, as a pain, as something sticky, as numbness, or as something nervous and shaking. Such blocks can surface anywhere in your body, from your throat, back, arms, legs, stomach, breasts, womb, vagina, knees, and hips.

Every part of your body reflects the way your consciousness functions in the physical world:

Your feet represent how grounded you are.

Your legs represent your ability to move forward.

Your hips reveal how flexible you are with change.

Your sexual palace refers to your intimate relationships and creativity.

Your stomach is linked to your sense of personal power.

Your back represents the past and support issues.

Your breasts express your ability to nourish.

Your heart is linked to giving and receiving love.

Your lungs reflect loneliness, grief and joy.

Your arms and hands represent your ability to get your creative ideas out into life.

Your throat and mouth relate to your ability to speak out.

Your eyes are connected to seeing the truth.

Your ears are connected to hearing the truth.

Your crown refers to your connection to the divine.

Of course, you have many more body parts and the list of how your awareness exists in your body goes on and on. Through practicing this technique, you discover that your body is always communicating with you to stay in alignment.

Next, focus on the area of your body that feels blocked, and then wait for the emotion or memory that has created that block to surface. You may feel an entanglement of different emotions. You may see a picture of a memory flash, you may receive a sense, or a knowing of how the blocked formed. Or, you may simply notice there is a block without any extra information. Just know that whatever is ready to come to the surface will, and the rest will wait for a more appropriate time. All is perfect.

2. Accept the Truth of Your Mud

The only way to truly release your mud is by welcoming and acknowledging all your emotions and the memories stored in them. You can no longer label certain emotions, feelings, or memories as bad, unacceptable, or wrong. Honor and accept what is there; then and only then will you will be able to feel the truth of why the block has formed inside your body.

The key here is to keep being present with the block until it begins to loosen, and as you do, hold a space of unconditional love—because this is ultimately what all blocks are after. Unconditional love is the ability to be nonjudgmental and completely compassionate. Unconditional love reminds you that you no longer have to repress parts of yourself, or hide, reject, shame, or deny them. Instead it allows you to be present in acceptance, and this is very healing for your mud. To allow your blocks to exist in the true reality of how they have formed is the premise of healing it. Without truth, greater truth cannot be revealed. This is a crucial component to ensure that your mud blossoms back to love. In order to truly heal, every part of you must be accepted and welcomed back to love.

Take care that you don't rush. Be present and patient with each block. As you are, the layers of emotions that create your mud will surface so you can acknowledge them. For example, you first may feel sadness; next anger will surface, followed by rage and disappointment. Each block will be embroiled in its own story and its own layering of emotions. Each layer will have formed for a different reason and may tell a different part of the story. Sometimes a block forms from one event, while at other times it could form from many events connected to the same trauma. Examples include heartbreak and relationship breakdowns beginning with your family and extending into your partnerships.

3. *Transform Your Mud.*

Your body is designed for transformation, and your sexual energy contains amazing healing properties. Just as you learned to express love through your body with your sexual energy in chapter six, you can also use this same process to clear your blocks and transform your mud. To begin, move your body and wake up the sexual force inside of you. You may want to dance, shaking and shimmying your hips. Such movements will help free and transform your blocks. On an inhale, squeeze your intimate muscles and use them like a pump to direct your sexual energy to the muddy area. Next, let your sexual energy connect to the love vibration under the block, and then on an exhale, intend your sexual energy and the love vibration to combine and direct them through the block to help it dissolve. Breathe your sexual energy through the lower vibrations and witness it dissolve. Repeat this a few times, moving your body in between to shake out the denser vibrations. As you go through this process, you will feel the layers of emotions, memories, and feelings surfacing; notice them, accept them, love them, and then give them freedom to transform into a new awareness. You will know the block has dissolved when you start to the feel the vibration of love flowing freely to that part of your body. This is an important part of the process, so keep sending your sexual energy and the vibration of love to that body part so the area can rejuvenate and return to health.

4. *Forgive Your Mud.*

You may notice that some blocks are stubborn and do not want to move. This requires forgiveness, a vital key in the transformation of all emotions. Forgiveness happens when you choose to stop suffering from events that have broken your heart. Abuse, betrayal, sexual assault, and abandonment become grievance stories that trap you in blaming the outside world. When you blame, you become a victim—relieving the negative experience over and over again. It takes skill to dismantle the pain and an even greater skill to become the heroine of your story rather than the victim. Forgiveness ushers in the compassion needed to melt the knots of negative emotions, and it brings wisdom to understand how they have formed. Forgiveness takes time, but every time you choose to forgive, you free yourself from being bound to past memories or other people's inadequacies. Forgiveness helps you to remember that you are worth more than what was imposed upon you. It offers separation and disconnect from that which does not honor the love inside of you. The ability to forgive is a virtue; it begins with you, then extends toward others. Through forgiveness you learn to return your mud to love.

The easiest way to forgive is to pretend that you are the great field of love looking down at your body and at the block you are trying to heal. From this perspective, you will be able to observe what and who needs to be forgiven, and most importantly why forgiveness is necessary. You may get insights and new awareness from the great field of love to solve your block. Throughout the process, visualize sending love to your body to help soften your thoughts, your body, and the block. This can be a very moving experience, one that will set you free so you can move forward in your life.

5. *Transcend Your Mud.*

Remember that every lower emotion within you wants to return to love. For example, broken love creates anger, but it can evolve into courage. Suppressed love creates sadness, but it can transform into joy. Rejected love creates unworthiness, but it can learn to remember its power. Uncertain love creates fear, but it can evolve into stability. Banished love creates loneliness, but it teaches self-love. Denied love creates jealousy, but it can promote more self-awareness. Every unbalanced emotion you have is pointing to a lesson of love you have not yet learned. Every bit of your mud, no matter how dark and twisted it may be, wants to return back to love—your job is to be present with it until it untangles.

The more you learn the lessons that love is trying to teach you, the more you will master life. For example, a sibling may have taken your share of an inheritance left by a parent. This would make you feel betrayed and vengeful, a feeling that could twist you in bitterness and hatred for years. The real lesson is knowing that your parents' love and care for you exists beyond the material gift left. By transcending into this awareness, the need for the physical gift disappears and a spiritual bridge of love is created between you and the loved one that has passed over; such a connection is more precious than any object.

Once you learn the lesson, you will notice a shift in your vibration. Your mind will feel clearer, your heart brighter, and your body energized. You will notice the relationships around you improving because you are choosing to interact in a more developed way. Keep questioning and intuiting the response of your emotions, where they come from, and why they have formed until you find resolution or a lesson of love. Every lesson will strengthen you with valuable insights that grant new ways to behave, respond, operate, and interact with life around you. This is how you change your reality because reality is only a reflection of who you are. Your ability to birth your mud through love allows you to recreate yourself as a higher vibrational being.

The key is to keep evolving into love so you can master your life. As you master this process, your ability to transform lower emotions into love will quicken. Instead of spending weeks lost in heartbreak and trapped in your mud, you will be able to fast-track your ability to process, learn, and transcend in minutes. This will make the evolution into love a fun and easy game. Every time you discover a lesson of love in your mud—celebrate! You may feel freer in your body, breathe easier, or experience relief and a sense that a weight has been released. This means that the mud within your consciousness, the mud that causes challenges within relationships or obstacles with your ambitions, has released. For this process it is essential that you also spend time reflecting how your lessons and new awareness can help you make better decisions, navigate through future situations with greater ease, and act in ways that are more appropriate for the benefit of all. Transcending your mud always requires you to reflect, learn your lesson, celebrate, and then use your new awareness to interact with life in a completely new way. These keys will ensure your evolution into the enlightenment of love.

Letting Love Pass Through You

Through your journey of transcending your lower emotions, you simultaneously learn to master the ability for love to pass through you. This means that your system has become refined enough to metabolize that which is not love and transform it into love. Through this ability your gift of healing awakens. This means that if you can do it for yourself, then you can also help others heal and transcend their own journey back to love. This could happen through a conversation, giving someone a hug, or just by walking into a room and letting your energy assist others to transform. The more you have healed within yourself, the clearer you will feel inside, and this in turn will ensure that your relationships are less dramatic. When you no longer operate from lower vibrational spaces that trigger your past traumas, you no longer trigger your partner to operate from those states either.

The ability to allow love to pass through you so that it can awaken another, makes the path of sensual enlightenment beautifully contagious. The love you generate ignites others to generate love. Even the smallest shift into the awareness of love can help to change the trajectory of another person's life. The flap of the butterfly wing in the southern hemisphere affects the weather in the northern hemisphere. Likewise, any time you emit love as an action, thought, or feeling, you educate life with new awareness. Letting love pass through you could be as faint as a breath or as intense as the release of a full-body orgasm. The more love you can allow to pass through your body, the more you discover yourself as your own soul mate. You are, after all, a woman in love who is discovering love through the self.

Reflection:

1. What lower emotion do you experienced the most? What experiences or memories have caused them?
2. What lower emotions do you hardly feel? Why do you think that is? What lessons have you learned not to feel those emotions?
3. Close your eyes and scan your body. Where do you feel your mud is? Where are the energy blocks and what do they feel like? What emotions and memories are stored there?
4. Go through the five-step process of "unlocking your mud" and record your findings. Which step was the easiest? Which was the most difficult and why? What lesson did you learn?
5. What does "letting love pass through you" mean to you?
6. What does it mean to be a woman in love who is discovering love through the self? How does this make you become your own soul mate?

9

You Are Your Own Soul Mate

To be your own soul mate means that you choose to love yourself more than anyone else can. You take responsibility for all of your own issues so you do not project dramas into the relationships around you. Self-love teaches you how to be kind to yourself so you can be more compassionate with others. It releases judgments, egoic needs, and demands that would otherwise jeopardize love. When you love yourself, your partner will be able to experience self-love too, and the generation and overflow of love will continue. Just as you may long for a partner to love every inch of you, you must first do this for yourself. Whatever you are needing from a partner, you are actually needing from yourself. You are the source of everything. Do you need approval? Approve of yourself. Do you need recognition? Then recognize your own brilliance. Do you want to be desired? Want and desire yourself! Do you want gifts and a vacation? Give yourself exactly that! If you have a need for love, love yourself so fully that love is all that you become. You are the "the one" you have been waiting for.

The more you love yourself, the more you will discover yourself. The dormant parts of you will awaken, and you can be who you truly are. And who you are is infinitely magnificent.

Gifted with Superpowers

Your ability to love yourself is your greatest superpower; from it stems an array of other superpowers to use, and we all know women have superpowers! In fact, most of us felt these superpowers as young girls. We felt a power that was in the core of our hearts, a potential that expressed itself as softness, wildness, beauty, passion, wisdom, rage, knowing, and truth. Every woman knows that the love inside of her is revolutionary and can blaze a path of transformation. Below are ten superpowers with which your feminine heart is gifted. As you read through them, allow the qualities to awaken in your heart.

1. *Kindness*

No other human quality will get you further in life than kindness. The quality of kindness teaches you how to be tender and compassionate, first with yourself and then with others. This approach is the most efficient way to transform the limitations that inhibit your aliveness. Kindness should never be perceived as weakness or vulnerability. Kindness has a strong and positive influence on others.

2. *Appreciation*

As a sensual, enlightened woman, you have learned to appreciate both yourself and others. By celebrating other people's accomplishments, you encourage them to grow. Secure in your own abilities, comparing yourself to others does not interest you. By appreciating others, you become inspired to be and do more, which of course bounces back and enables others to appreciate you. Love flows through appreciation.

3. Elegance

Elegance is grace expressed through appearance, movements, personal style, and behavior. Elegance is a sophisticated dignity that radiates from you when you refine who you truly are. An elegant woman never copies or compares; she is only and always herself. By holding good posture, your energy has a mystery, a softness, a strength, and a cleverness to it. When you possess elegance, you are graceful even in the midst of a challenge. You are able to handle yourself in a noble and ethical manner. Elegance encourages others to respect and honor you.

4. Composure

Composure is the beauty of self-control. Without a sense of composure, conflicting situations and relationships can create chaos. When you have composure, you understand the concept of *less equals more*. The less you react, defend, explain, become fearful or controlling, the more command you have over a situation. Composure allows you to stand tall in the face of loss or challenge. It also allows you to maintain a quiet and wise stillness. It promotes peace.

5. Courage

Courage is the willingness to dare greatly in your life. It takes courage to love fully, to change yourself when necessary, to feel deeply, to chase your dreams with passion, and to leave a relationship when it no longer works. To become courageous, you must fearlessly identify and push through your limitations. A courageous heart sees the highest vision and obtains it regardless of the obstacles. A courageous heart is strong.

6. Empowerment

When you are self-loving, you naturally possess a quiet confidence that empowers you to be more of your authentic self. Empowerment brings self-awareness and dedication to self-development and personal growth. It provides the knowledge and confidence needed to succeed. Empowerment brings the attitude that positive things will always happen. It also allows you to be clear and persistent about who you are, the direction of your ambitions, and what you need from relationships to be happy. An empowered life is not based on pretenses; instead, it is a direct reflection of your authentic self. Empowerment allows you to be strong, confident, tender, wise, and passionate all at once.

7. Longing

The feminine heart is by nature a longing heart. In the depth of longing, there will never be satisfaction unless you find a way to honor and share your creative self. You might think you lack this or that, but your yearnings and longings are only expressions of a deeper need—the desire to radiate who you truly are. When longing is celebrated, it can become the greatest gift. So take a risk: if you long for more honesty, BE honest. If you long for more power, BE powerful.

A longing to "experience yourself completely," go "deeper," and be fulfilled is a longing with no end; it is infinite. As a woman, you must learn to channel who you are into this world as a way of becoming, not as a way of giving yourself away or getting something in return. It means that you share who you are from the very source of your soul; longing is the pull that will help you discover who you truly are in this world.

8. Intelligence

The heart of a woman is sublimely intelligent with knowledge, intuition, and emotional maturity. Intelligence is a creative, practical, and well-informed energy that shows you how to turn obstacles into opportunities. It teaches you to be practical and utilize the resources already available to enhance and upgrade your life. A woman's intelligence also gives her the ability to process information through the filter of love, bringing profound wisdom that cannot be taught or studied.

9. Honesty

Every woman knows that people gravitate toward what is real. This is achieved by being simple, up front, gentle, and with direct communication. Honesty allows others to trust that you have no ulterior motives. When you are relationship-oriented versus agenda-oriented, there is no need to change who you are depending on who you are with. There is no need to manipulate a situation because you are empowered. An honest heart is one that is aligned to love.

10. *Wildness*

Wildness means being unrestricted and free. It honors the passion that bubbles up or explodes within, and it cares nothing for rules. The only conviction of a wild heart is following your intuition and experiencing life until your authentic self is awakened. A wild heart is adventurous and very free. Sparked with creation energy, it is a quality that enlivens and rejuvenates any situation. A wild heart grants every woman the freedom to be more.

All of these superpowers require self-love. The more you embody them, the more illuminated you will become. This will make you glow better than any bronzer you can buy. When you are in love with yourself, beauty is no longer a commodity; it becomes a permanent state of being.

Beauty Is Not a Commodity—It Is a Frequency

Beauty by definition is a quality that gives intense pleasure. Beauty can be revealed in the sound of laughter, a smile, or the vibrant color of a flower. Beauty shows itself through kindness. Beauty is soft, graceful, and electrifying to the touch. Beauty has an exquisite presence, and when we connect to it and fall into it, even for a moment, we fall in love. Beauty allows us to feel love and live from the heart. Beauty opens a pathway to divinity, enabling your heart to connect with the frequency of heaven. If you allow yourself to expand every moment of beauty, you are showered with love continually. The heavens have found a portal to radiate through you.

'There are a thousand ways to beautify the life around you.'

Beauty is a state of being. It is not attached to having to be beautiful; it just is. Beauty is a way of being, a way of feeling, a way of seeing yourself and life around you. Beauty is a frequency we choose to tune into just like a radio station. Beauty allows us to activate love in our heart. It is one of our feminine superpowers. We can feel it, smell it, hear it, taste it, and know it. There are thousands of ways to beautify the life around you: in your home, in your relationships, by seeing the beauty in others, in washing the dishes, or by discovering your beautiful body while in the shower.

Because women are hungry—and dare I say, *starving*—for more beauty in their lives, beauty has become a commodity, full of big companies selling us so-called beauty products. Instead of acknowledging our abilities to create beauty, we buy into the drama of not smelling right, believing wrinkles are ugly, or there is weight to lose. By disliking our bodies, we feel diminished and powerless, and we succumb to the next product instead of invoking the frequency of love in our lives. The more we feel insecure and unconfident, the less we feel beautiful. Take time to educate yourself so you can make empowered choices. Learn to see through the marketing campaigns of "beauty" products.

'When a woman takes ownership of her beauty,
her beauty is no longer a regime.'

When a woman takes ownership of her beauty, her beauty is no longer a regime. Beauty becomes a divine ritual. She finds the pleasure and the joy in her beauty by being unique. Take care of your beauty as an act of reverence and a tribute to your inner radiance. Tend to your beauty not as a way of conforming or copying but as an act of expressing the divine within you. Your beauty practices are a way of honoring and tending to the temple of the soul—your body.

Now when you adorn your body temple with jewelry, bright red nails, high heels, hair color, and makeup, do it because it is delightful, a celebration of yourself—not because you have been told to wear a mask, believing that your authentic self is not "beautiful" enough. The next time you dress or put on makeup, beautify the dialogue you have with yourself. You might say to yourself:

"Wow, I look good."

"My hips look great with these shoes."

"My eyes are magnetizing."

Be in awe of yourself as you paint and dress to accentuate the beauty that is you. This act of self-love is natural for the sensual, enlightened woman.

When a woman loves herself, her face no longer shows exhaustion, anger, or disappointment. Her skin softens with self-love, and her life frustrations do not crinkle and crease her skin. No longer will she be burdened by life, because the freedom in her heart gives her a youth that no anti-wrinkle cream can offer. The sensually enlightened woman knows that the combination of her sexual energy and the love existing within her cells is the perfect antiaging formula.

Ten-Minute Antiaging Rejuvenation Exercise - *refer to figure 11:*

1. Every night before you go to sleep, lie on your back. Do some deep breathing until you feel every muscle in your body and face relax. Inhale and breathe love in from the universe. Exhale any stress, anger, or tensions that your cells are holding. As you do this, you may feel memories of the day leaving your body and mind. Some memories will free your body from negative energies; other memories may brighten you with positive energy. Repeat until you feel your heart center and your body flowing with love.

2. Now place your hands on your heart center and feel you palms filling with love. Next, bathe your body in the love that comes from your heart. This includes your fingers, arms, shoulders, neck, breasts, waist, hips, legs, and toes. As you caress your skin, notice that you are opening up your energy pathways to start flowing with love. You may also notice your sexual energy beginning to activate in your sexual palace and the erogenous zones of your body. As this occurs, you may begin to feel your body blessing you with beautiful orgasmic or pleasurable sensations. If you would like to deepen this experience, use the rest of the blossoming techniques that you learned in chapter six, *The Art Of Blossoming.*

3. Next move to your face. Gently caress your every part of your face: your eyes, nose, ears, cheeks, lips. As you do this, invite the love that exists within the cells of your face to release and blossom. You also may want to use the tips of your fingertips and apply light pressure to stimulate the face in new ways.

4. Now focus on your intimate muscles. Squeeze and use them like a pump to bring your sexual energy up to your face. As

you inhale, squeeze, smile, and direct your sexual energy up through your heart center into your face. As you exhale, allow your loving sexual energy to blossom through the cells of your face. Keep repeating this movement, but each time you inhale, focus your attention on a specific area, such as your cheeks or forehead. Make sure you include your neck and chin area as well.

5. If there are other areas of your body that you would like to beautify—your hips or stomach, for example—then you can apply the same process to them.

6. When you're ready, you can fall asleep with your face and body glowing. The more you do this, the more you will awaken to start your day with a radiating glow of youthful vitality.

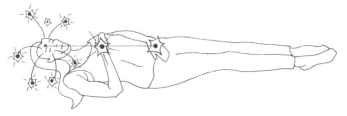

Figure 11: Anti Aging Rejuvenation Exercise

Celebrate Being 'In Love' With Love

The more you celebrate your unique beauty, the more you will celebrate your true self. This is key to becoming your own soul mate. Vibrating self-love is super attractive, and since like attracts like, love will materialize into physical reality and magnetize soul mates for you to exchange with. Exchanging your unique frequency of love with another person will allow you to experience a version of love that has never occurred before. You, beautiful woman, live in a world of hearts, and therefore you live in a world with infinite versions of love to explore. Remember your soulmates are simply an expression of yourself. As you awaken to your authentic self, the perfect mate or mates will arise as mirror manifestation of who and what you are. This also includes the limitations that both of you need to evolve out of. Although union with another is super fulfilling, finding your soulmate is not the ultimate experience. From the enlightened position you are removing the barriers, illusions and blocks to the realization that you are always one with love. This then makes the union with love the ultimate fulfillment. From here, lonely feelings melt as you realize that love links you to everyone and everything. At the deepest level, everything and everyone is your soul mate—there is only "one."

Reflection:

1. What does it mean to be your own soul mate?
2. What can you do to love yourself more?
3. Which superpower of the female heart do you feel you have mastered?
4. Which superpower of the female heart do you feel is lacking? What can you do to embody it?
5. Which superpower excites you the most? Why?
6. How can you turn your beauty regime into a ritual?
7. Why does a joyful heart make you more youthful?
8. Why is it important to fall in love with yourself first, and then others?

10

A World Of Hearts

"A soulmate is someone who has locks that fit our keys, and keys to fit our locks. When we feel safe enough to open the locks, our truest selves step out and we can be completely and honestly who we are." —Richard Bach

Deep within is the need to find the one person who can truly open our locks. The one who makes us tingle and feel alive, the one who understands the deepest parts of ourselves, the one to share the journey of life with. We all desire someone who can give us love and help us learn to love in return. A soul mate comes in many forms and can come into our lives for one day or stay for twenty years or more. They come to awaken us, bringing keys to help us understand the multifaceted nature of love.

Soul mates exchange the information of love through touch, words, experiences, and sometimes tragedies. It is through this exchange that one masters love. The mastery of love brings true love. True love is what many refer to as unconditional love—a state that is free from negativity, drama, judgment, or lack. True love is supportive, nurturing, liberating, emotionally intelligent, kind, generous, evolving, and magical. True love is the desire to master all the virtues of love with another person. When two people love themselves, both parties overflow with love for each other, and this is a beautiful moment. True love is the ability to uplift your partner in love.

Mastering love is the main purpose of human life. We are here to gain the wisdom of love, learn the power of love, feel affection, get swept away by romance, be ignited by passion, develop friendships that are truthful and loyal, learn compassion, and understand how to become selfless. These qualities are taught to us by our soul mates, and the lessons come in different forms. They come from lovers, partners, family members, and friends; they come from a brief meeting with a stranger or from our pets, and even from the sun, stars, and nature around us.

Mastering Love Through Connection

We learn to master love through every interaction we have with others. Every person that crosses your path will teach you something valuable about the virtues of love. Sometimes they will bring you insights, and other times they will make you aware of how love can be corrupted. Both are valuable lessons, for in order to truly become aware of the truth, we also need to become aware of that which distorts the truth. Those that teach as about love are our soul mates. A soul mate is not limited to being your romantic partner; it could be anyone with whom you choose to experience a facet of love. It could be your mother, your child, your sibling, your friend, a brief meeting with a stranger, or your pet animal. These types of connections help create the experience for you to practice exchanging and honoring love. In the highest version, a soul mate would apply the virtues of love to ensure that the relationship dynamic always returns to a place of harmony. Whereby enough heightened awareness has been generated for both parties to reveal more of their authentic self.

'The authentic self is really your unique version of love.'

The authentic self is really your unique version of love, and as you develop, your unique version of love will also evolve. You will continue to refine your desires, opinions, perceptions, tastes, and preferences as you master yourself as your own soul mate. To be authentic means that you operate first from your truth and then simultaneously accept another person's truth. To do this requires total acceptance of yourself and other person, the courage not to be swayed out of your truth, the ability for both of you to communicate your needs, the wisdom to create solutions if incongruencies arise, and the sheer joy, spontaneity, creativity, and freedom that love offers to spark a more sublime connection. True love occurs between two soul mates when both can generate an excess of self-love that overflows to the other person and raises them to higher consciousness. This process can be never-ending, resulting in both parties becoming so united that they become one love operating from two bodies. This experience can extend out to include family members, friends, other lovers or romantic partners, and ultimately all of humanity. The ancient Chinese proverb knows this truth: "When there is light in the soul, there is light in the family, when there is light in the family there is light in the nation, when there is light in the nation, there is light in the world." We may still have a long way to go as a collective society, but the journey always begins with being your own soul mate first. Only then can it progress to include others.

Conversely, in the lowest version of soul mate connections, the values of love are continuously undermined and broken, with neither partner having the skills to generate self-love. Instead, the lack of love demands that each partner supply what the other requires, leading to codependent and dysfunctional relationships. Misinterpretation and miscommunication of one's needs develop, projections occur that trap each other in distorted perceptions, and resentments arise when the love given is not up to "standard." To further compound the disharmony, ego demands, narcissistic wounds, unresolved childhood traumas, and family, societal, or religious obligations can imprison one and cause them to behave against their truth. This further inhibits both parties to discover their authentic selves, which then denies the application of the virtues of love that are required to bring both healing to self and the relationship. Such soul mate relationships are filled with toxic emotions, tensions, arguments, hurts, criticisms, abuse, jealousy, possessiveness, control, manipulation, and lots of heartbreak and hurt feelings. Other red flags are if your partner constantly denies, criticizes, or dismisses you, constantly tests your boundaries, refuses to talk through issues, are overly critical about their previous partners, you get a gut feeling there is something wrong, or you justify their bad behaviour. Sometimes these types of soul mate connections occur, not by conscious or willing choice but because of family obligations, the pull of sexual chemistry, by perceived pressures that require each person to "check" boxes such as get married or have a family, or simply from the desperate need to have a relationship even if it is toxic.

Whatever the reason for connection, all toxic soul mate connections have one thing in common—they all bring to the surface the corrupted versions of love both parties have inside. From here you have three choices: 1) choose to heal together, 2) step away from the relationship and heal, or 3) continue the connection knowing that it will remain toxic. However, if you choose the third option, you will eventually conclude that you need to step away and heal, and this is a super empowering moment. This is the moment where, regardless of the issues and the traumas you have inside, the desire to return to the love that exists inside of you is greater. Every low-vibration soul mate connection also reveals to you the pain and the disharmony that gets created when love is broken. This is a highly valuable lesson; you will not be able to protect and promote the integrity of love unless you understand the chaos that gets created when it does not exist. It is of the highest value that you intentionally heal the corruptions that you have experienced; through this process, you learn to return every disharmony back to harmony. This will then become a highly prized asset in mastering love for future relationships.

This world is filled with duality, and no matter how much you can generate your own self-love and apply the lessons of love to evolve all of your relationships, you will always cross paths with those that don't. The difference is that instead of being pulled into the drama of corrupted love, you will be able to discern the parameters and choose the appropriate interaction so that you pass through the connection without being harmed. Sometimes it will be a simple "no thank you" that avoids the connection, and other times due to circumstances such as work or family connections, you will discover how to avoid reacting to others' bad behavior, or you will take the appropriate action when the person chooses to operate in a more balanced way. This diplomatic skill definitely takes practice to master because those we love tend to trigger our inadequacies the most. But love is such a refined energy, that in order to truly master it, you will be presented with relationships that reflect your limitations. This is so you can refine your concept of love within. Welcome to the world of hearts, beautiful woman, a sometimes painful but nonetheless glorious experience of journeying into love via human relationships. Remember, the ultimate key to this journey is to heal your distorted concepts of love first, learn to love yourself more than anyone else can, and always remember that the greatest love connection you will ever truly have is with love itself.

'The greatest love connection you will always have is with love itself.'

The most intense forms of soul mate connections are those that create sexual chemistry. Since your sexual energy is an ever-evolving force, you will find yourself attracted to different types of men and women at different times of your life. This is because sexual energy always seeks connection, and when the sexual energy of two soul mates collide, the spark that fuels intimate desire begins. Such a connection arouses both parties to find and explore the other person.

In the highest form, sexual energy seeks out the love vibration in your partner, and vice versa. Through this meeting your essence will light each other up, giving the feeling that you have been "found". A sense of renewal follows as each party's sexual energy helps birth the other into existence. This experience can only exist when both parties have learned to be their own soul mate and can cultivate their own sexual energy to unite with their heart. From this stance, one's sexual energy has learned to sublimate from being a physical force to a more refined version that desires to experience exchange as opposed to gratification.

In the lowest form, sexual energy will seek intimacy that does not center around loving exchange and authentic relating. Instead it desires the other person to grant physical satisfaction. This kind of union often makes you feel used and taken advantage of. You feel that you have given in to another person's desires in order to experience "love"—you sense that they may want your body but not necessarily *you*. A manipulation occurs, making you believe that love exists when self-gratification is the reality.

Sexual energy is such a powerful force that if one has not learned how to sublimate it, it creates some very interesting relationship dynamics. Passionate love is exciting, but crazy love can be very destructive, leading to heartbreak or another "failed relationship." This cycle is very common and can lead someone to give up on love or become too broken to return a relationship back to love. You always have the choice, however, to walk away and not play out another person's drama.

The Key to Feeling Empowered in Relationships

In order to feel empowered in relationships, you must unite your sexual energy with your heart first. This connection—which I refer to as the "divine inner marriage"—will stabilize your need to be supplied with love and sexual energy by the other person. (You can find a recorded meditation on this to help you in my FREE *Rebirth Into Love* Online course. Go to www.vanyasilverten.com to locate it.)

A woman's body is receptive in nature, and deep within we have a longing to be filled with love and empowered by sexual energy. Since at the core of our being, we women are romantics, we subconsciously desire someone else to complete us. But often, that desire turns into a desperate need, that becomes so overpowering, that any sense of guiding intuition or discernment is overlooked. This often leads one to choose inappropriate relationships to fill the void within, or there is an inability to let go of a relationship when it's over, or in worst cases, it can lead to obsessions that you cannot control. When a woman's sexual energy fills her heart, and her heart energy overflows to fill her sexual palace with love, she will complete herself and therefore will not require someone else to complete her. Instead she will seek a partner to share life with. This alignment inside a woman's body is the first step to healing broken love patterns within relationships. Without it, a woman will misjudge her partner because she is operating from a place of lack. In extreme cases this can cause the victim mentality we often see in abusive situations. A sensually enlightened woman operates from a place of fulfillment and abundance. This then gives her the power to stand in her authentic self and always express her truth.

When the sexual energy supports the heart chakra, you will be less likely to be taken advantage of sexually by another person, and you won't feel the loss if your advances are rejected. This is true on the romantic level, but it can also extend to other interactions, including self-promotion and business dealings. After my sexual energy had learned to sublimate through my body, I became confident to claim myself as a professional healer. I increased my hourly rate, got over my social media phobia, could negotiate with more confidence, and was unaffected by literacy agents rejecting my book concepts. The more powerful I felt by my own energy, the more power I had to command my life. The more love stabilized within me, the more abundance I was able to experience in my everyday life. It was as though I had no choice but to create a better life for myself. Ideas would flood my mind, inspiration would open my heart, and the sheer excitement of creating a better life willed me into action. The journey of realizing my life purpose also deepened my relationship with myself. I cared for myself better, used encouraging self dialogue instead of criticism, and lived in celebration because I could finally be proud of who I was.

> *'As a woman, you are designed to feel powerful*
> *in every situation you find yourself in.'*

You are also designed to be filled with love and overflowing with a sense of fulfilment and abundance. The cherry of course, is to have this replicated in your relationships.

Your soul will invite a relationship into your life for three main reasons. The first is to experience and master love through harmonizing with another person. The second is to highlight the distorted love within each other and find the wisdom to heal it. The third is to love yourself more than anyone else can. In order to achieve this, you often have many different types of relationships to ensure that these dynamics play out. Relationships form in an infinite amount of ways, and the dynamics within are equally as complex. Let's explore them . . .

Soul Mates Everywhere

Some soul mate relationships last for a certain period of time to close a karmic chapter. Other relationships are meant to bear children, but the partners are not necessarily meant to remain together. Some relationships are just plain confusing because a melting pot of emotions develop. These types of relationships usually teach us to love ourselves first.

The more quickly you can identify what type of soul mate experience you are having with whom, the more gracefully you will learn your lessons of love. Problems arise if you misjudge the reason someone has come into your life or project onto them a certain role they are not meant to fulfill. Every relationship teaches you valuable lessons that you can use to enhance your future relationships. Often soul mates appear in disguise. You might not be physically attracted to them when you first meet them, but there is a mysterious force that tells you to "go and explore."

The first time I met my husband, we did not hit it off romantically. Initially I put him into the friend zone, but as the weeks rolled by, I became curious about him, his culture, his upbringing, and his thoughts about life. Although I felt he would be a great partner for a long-term relationship, I was too concerned with my budding singing career. I did not want to be distracted, so we stayed as friends. Over the next few months, I noticed that every day at work, I would see a woman wearing a heart on her necklace. Everyday a different woman, wearing a different heart necklace, would come into the busy health shop I managed. There were gold hearts, stone hearts, gem hearts, wooden hearts, blue hearts, pink hearts, and many more types of hearts. I finally got the message that the universe wanted me to be with this man, and so it is.

Below are several types of relationship categories to help you navigate the ocean of love. You may find some soul mates that have come into your life have played out more than one role, or that a relationship has evolved from one role to the next, and you may also get clues of how to evolve the relationship to experience deeper and longer lasting love. Or you may notice that your partner played out one role, and you were playing out another role, thus creating a mismatch in your connection. It is always important to identify the type of relationship the connection offers, as this will help you to master love easily and effortlessly. Since the types of soul mate experiences available are infinite, the list below is not definitive. As you journey through your path of love, you may be able to identify more.

1. *Soul Mate*

A soul mate is anyone who crosses your path to teach you valuable lessons about what love is and what love it not. This could be a lover, a friend, your mother, father, your children, siblings, work colleagues, or even your pet dog or cat. A soul mate will light you up, and there is a sense of familiarity or a knowing that you have met before. Usually there is an energetic connection that magnetizes you both or an urge to discover the other person more. An exchange of energy, ideas, and experiences will take place. Soul mates often have the missing information that completes one another. Since we have a lot of missing information, we often need many soul mate connections to gain all of it. The saying "It takes a village to raise a child" is true for your entire life. In this case, it takes a tribe of soul mates to raise you in love and abundance - your soul family.

2. Your Soul Family

These people come into your life and usually are of no genetic relationship, but they care for you like family. Often we outgrow our genetic family dynamic and are in need of those who are in alignment to our truth. When you meet a soul family member, you feel as though you have met before or that you know them. There will be care, friendship, and support from your soul family. You will usually meet to help encourage each other to master life.

3. Your Own Soul Mate

To be your own soul mate means that you choose to love yourself more than anyone else can. It ensures that you take responsibility for all of your own issues, so you do not project dramas in the relationships around you. Self-love teaches you how to be kind to yourself so you can be more compassionate with others. It releases judgments, egoic needs, and demands that would otherwise jeopardize love. When you love yourself, your partner will love themselves, and the generation and overflow of love continues.

4. Flirt/Fling

These relationships are not long-term. A flirt or fling could be as quick as a cup of coffee with someone, or a two-week romance during a holiday. They bring a new wave of love to you and remind you that love does exist. They often act as a carrot to entice you out of the situation you are in. Sometimes they come to awaken you out of a lonely place, or to stimulate a stagnant relationship that needs to change. These usually prepare you for your next relationship so you can experience love at a deeper level.

5. Ego Mates

Ego mates are concerned with whether the other person makes them "look" good. Energetically they wrap their ego around their partner. They like their partners to do the right things, behave the right ways, go to the right places, hang out with the right people, wear the right clothes, live in the right houses, have the right career, and earn the right income. They are conditional, superficial, and material status is the driver, not love. Most ego relationships are transitory, coming and going as partners make each other feel better about themselves—or not. Ego mates look outside the relationship for fulfillment. As a result, these relationships are prone to cheating or continually looking for a better relationship.

6. Karmic Soul Mates

Karmic soul mates come together specifically for the purpose of teaching or working out an issue. They have unfinished business or a shared trauma or need. This could range from their souls agreeing to have a child together but not necessarily stay in the relationship or, having a relationship that clashes with arguments until kind communication is learned. Karmic mates are sometimes difficult or challenging, but they don't have to be. When a relationship is difficult, it is because we are refusing to acknowledge something in ourselves; we have healing to do. When we accept this wisdom, we can move the relationship into a better place. In a karmic relationship, you have to work through the issues; otherwise you will keep attracting the same relationships over and over again.

7. Bad Apples

Bad apple relationships are unhealthy. They might look good to begin with, but at the core there is something rotten and destructive. Such connections can be manipulative, controlling, and abusive—physically, emotionally, mentally, spiritually, and sexually. These relationships leave you feeling confused, rejected, unworthy, angry, victimized, and lonely.

In worst cases, the lack of love creates a more desperate need to receive love from the abuser. Oftentimes one partner will deny or readjust their truth, believing in the other's lies and manipulations to receive a scrap of love. Over time this will corrupt and distort the person's sense of self, often to the point where he or she will forget they can generate their own love. In the worst cases, someone can get so accustomed to corrupted love that they will begin to create bad apple relationships themselves.

No one should ever be in an abusive relationship, and if you are in one, then you must leave, even if you have children. Bad apple relationships will not change, no matter how much a person promises. You have to muster strength and conviction in yourself so you can leave the negative partnership. Then you must heal and go on a self-love journey before you enter in a new relationship. Under no circumstances should you let yourself be a victim to an abuser; nor should you be tempted to rescue the one who keeps corrupted love. It's their responsibly to evolve and heal themselves, not yours.

8. *Narcissists*

Narcissists cannot think beyond their own paradigm because they are in love with their "idealized" image of themselves. Many times they will project their perfect self through conversations and arguments to avoid being seen as the real disenfranchised, wounded self. Since they are consumed with themselves, they have little awareness of your personal or emotional needs and instead will require you to support their needs and emotions. If something goes wrong in the relationship, it will be your fault, and if something goes wrong in their life, it will be your fault as well. Although they may come across as having a strong personality, underneath their armor is a lot of vulnerability that swings between an inferiority and a superiority complex. This imbalance makes them hypersensitive or defensive when they feel they are being challenged. Then this will make you feel like you are "walking on eggshells" as you try to adjust yourself to accommodate their needs.

These types of relationships will often make you feel heartbroken because you will be unable to authentically relate or exchange each other's truth to evolve the relationship. Furthermore, a narcissist has an inability to love themselves, because they choose to deny the lower feelings of rejection that lives within them. Instead you will find yourself being the one rejected on a daily basis. Although not ideal, you will be able function in a mild narcissistic relationship if you do not expect to be validated or to "share" all areas of life with them. The key here, as always, is to have the relationship with yourself that you cannot have with your partner, and then fall in love with life so that every sunset is magical with or without them.

9. Addicts

Being in a relationship with an addict can be extremely heartbreaking, especially if you were with them prior to their addiction. An addiction could include drugs, alcohol, cigarettes, shopping, gambling, sex, or eating, and range from emotional, mental, and physical addiction. These types of relationships will always make you feel as if there are three people in the relationship, and you are not the priority. How functional your relationship with them can be is dependent on the severity of the addiction. There may be lying, cheating, stealing, deception, and manipulation so they can continue to fuel their habit. As a result, relationships are usually the first components of an addict's life to be destroyed. Those that do stay in a relationship with an addict, might believe their love can fix or cure them. The reality is that all that you can do is motivate them to get treatment. Those that choose to stay in a relationship with an addict will need to set strong boundaries, and if the addict doesn't adhere to them, the healthy option is to then end the relationship. Luckily for the addict that does seek treatment, the relationship can often be salvaged. The worst-case scenario is if the other partner starts using the same substance as a way to "bond" with the addict or enable them with the substance to remain in the relationship with you.

10. Codependent Relationships

Codependent relationships are created when one or more partners lack self-esteem and look for a relationship for validation. We usually learn this type of behavior from watching and imitating other family members relate in similar ways. Although a codependent has good intentions, they often take on a martyr's role, becoming the "benefactor" to the other's person's needs. The codependent will repeatedly try to rescue their partner and may begin to make excuses or overcompensate for their partner's bad behavior. In the worst cases, they allow their partner to continue on a destructive course (such as addictions or abuse), and this then allows them to become more reliant on their unhealthy caretaking. The codependent experiences a sense of reward and satisfaction for being "needed." However, when caretaking becomes compulsive, the codependent will end up feeling helpless and like a victim but is often unable to break the cycle of behavior. Codependents are attracted to the weakness they feel inside themselves with others, which keeps spiraling into destructive and needy behavior.

Characteristics of Codependent People:

- An exaggerated sense of responsibility for the actions of others
- A tendency to confuse love and pity, with the tendency to "love" people they can feel sorry for and rescue
- A tendency to always do more than their share
- A tendency to become hurt when people don't recognize their efforts
- An unhealthy dependence on relationships. The codependent will do anything to hold on to a relationship and avoid the feeling of abandonment
- An extreme need for approval and recognition
- A sense of guilt when asserting themselves
- A compelling need to control others
- Lack of trust in self and others
- Fear of being abandoned or alone
- Difficulty identifying feelings
- Rigidity or difficulty adjusting to change
- Problems with intimacy and boundaries
- Chronic anger
- Lying and dishonesty
- Poor communications
- Difficulty making decisions

11. *Crazy Love*

This type of relationship is like being on a never-ending rollercoaster. Filled with passion, chemistry, romance, arguments and misunderstandings. Crazy love mates are often caught in the tension of love versus hate. Regular breaks ups and reunions are normal, where sexual intimacy becomes the medicine that creates peace between partners. Both partners genuinely care and love the other, but they also get deeply triggered and hurt by the other, and this leads to revenge and retaliation. Crazy love is a fiery dynamic that can feel very alive, the key is to develop excellent communication skills, so the passion does not turn into destruction.

12. Play Mates

These relationships are purely for enjoyment. There are no expectations and there is no destined futured. Play mates are absolutely for enjoying the moment and teach each other how to be truthful, present and spontaneous. Usually filled with laughter and adventure, these types of relationships help make the ordinary extraordinary.

13. Stale Mates

Stale mates are those relationships that need to end, but neither party is bold enough to make the move. In these relationships, the spark has gone and there is little or no conversation. Perhaps it's because they have outgrown each other, or so much resentment has built up between them that a repulsion is created. Maybe neither partner has a desire to spark each other with new life. You may notice a stale mate relationship at a restaurant where a couple is dining without conversation. Both people stare off into the distance and are merely going through the motions of eating. People in a stale mate relationship can live years and years in this state, neither one growing because both are choosing to live in stagnation for fear of change.

14. The Rebound

Rebounds occur after a significant relationship has ended and you fill the emptiness in your life with another person. This type of connection is usually short-lived due to one partner's emotional instability and the desire to distract themselves from a painful breakup. In these relationships, either you are on the rebound or you are your partner's rebound. There may be lots of conversation and comparison about past partners, as the rebounder tries to remold the present relationship to their past one. The key here is to always take your time and heal you own heart first, processing the relationship you have been in, where it didn't work, where it did, how you grew, what you learned. This process will help you gain insights about how to enter into a true relationship (not a rebound) in a more masterful way.

15. The Player

Players are people who are just after a sexual or intimate relationship with you. They know exactly how to get you aroused so you will say yes to their advances. They give you attention, they say the right things, they touch you in the right places, and before you know it, you are intimate with them. At certain times in your journey to mastering love and your sexuality, this can be a good experience if you knew the experience was purely physical with no expectations of an ongoing relationship. Such an experience may make you feel empowered as a woman that can enjoy her sexuality without giving her heart away. If you have not mastered this, though, you will most likely feel that you have been used or taken advantage of after being intimate with them. A player usually enjoys you once or twice and then moves on to the next game.

16. The Fraud

These relationships are too good to be true or as my great granny would say 'too sweet to be wholesome.' They often begin like a whirlwind romance filled with compliments, affection and even talks of marriage in the first weeks of meeting. He or she may come across as very confident, wealthy and successful. You may even feel like you have found the perfect life partner. The aim of the fraud is to make you fall in love so that you become blind to their true intentions. The cracks will begin to appear when the fraud needs urgent money for an unexpected problem, or pressures you to marry them in order to stay in the country or wants you to sign over your possessions like your car or house. It may start with small requests and then build to larger ones. Their 'love' and affection becomes conditional, but you may not notice because you have been tricked into being unconditionally in love with them.

17. *One Sided Love*

Sometimes you may meet someone that lights you up so much, that you feel you are meant to be together. You may experience gushes of love when you are near them, and even get the feeling that there is a magnetic pull of attraction between you both. Except when you go to confess your love to him/her, they reply that they do not feel the same way. Then you are left feeling very confused because that person felt so right for you. The reasons why someone may not return love are complex, and it's ok for someone not to love you when you love them. The key is not to feel rejected or try to convince them to love you. Instead use it as an opportunity to notice that there are people in this world who will light you up without a relationship ever developing.

18. *Companion Mates*

These are souls who have agreed to enjoy a warm and loving long-term relationship. They share their lives for specific reasons, such as raising children or expanding their understanding of genuine love. They can last a lifetime and are characterized by respect, affection, intimacy, commitment, safety, and loyalty. They don't ignore the ups and downs of life; instead they have agreed to navigate them together. Their love grows deeper and blossoms over time, but it is still possible for companion mates to grow apart as each follows their individual path, thus turning their deep care and love for each other into a lifelong friendship.

19. *Lovers/Tantric Flame*

These soul mate connections can be completely sexually igniting. There is deep care, sensitivity, and arousal between partners. Usually these connections occur on a deeply physical yet very spiritual level. They may or may not develop into relationships, but the sexual exchange can be very healing for both partners. Touch, connection, and intimacy are powerfully liberating. No words are needed; no promises are made; no obligations or expectations are set. These soulmate connections are designed to help you experience sexual love in a very physical, body-orientated way. You melt into each other, you exchange soul energies, and you rebirth each other into a brighter, more complete experience of life.

20. *Soul Flame/Twin Flame*

Once you meet a soul flame, your life will change forever. There is usually a very strong magnetic attraction and recognition that you have been waiting for them your entire life. You feel a sense of expansion with them as they help to move you beyond your limited reality. They are aligned to your soul, but they are also sent to challenge, awaken, and stir different parts of you in order to transcend to a higher level of consciousness and awareness. Once the lessons have been learned, physical separation can occur. This connection is multifaceted, and a soul flame can be your friend, lover, teacher, muse, and nurturer all at once. The key to a soul flame is that they remind you of who you truly are because they reflect your highest truth. They can come into your life for a day, a week, or a lifetime.

21. *Cosmic Flame*

You can have a cosmic flame relationship with any being or energy beyond the human realm. This could include the sun, moon, trees, a sacred site, a beautiful star in the sky, or an angelic force. It's similar to the experience of a soul flame, except that a relationship does not develop in the physical world. It is a psychic, telepathic, and energetic connection that occurs through the ethers. For example, it can occur from sunlight shining down on your body and activating a deeper sense of self to awaken. In such cases the sun is coded with information that is missing in the receiver. There can be rushes of energy through the body as your vessel upgrades its vibration to embody more of the higher self. Teachings about the truth of one's soul purpose is often downloaded. The purpose of a cosmic soul flame is to provide you with the missing information needed to upgrade your awareness about yourself and life. They often provide the spiritual wisdom that cannot be received from human relationships.

22. *True Love*

To be in a relationship where both people love themselves and are able to complete themselves makes a partnership powerful, passionate, and purposeful. No one operates out of obligations or has to fill the emotional needs of the other. No one has to deny who they are or live in silent resentment because they are too afraid to speak their truth. No one says nasty things to the other person or manipulates them to gain power. When two people love themselves, the relationship is healthy and vibrant. There is joy and acceptance, freedom and care, mystery and support. These types of relationships are dynamic and empowering. They are filled with wisdom and playfulness. Both partners can be fluid and open to the changing needs of the other. There is a genuine desire to support the other person to become who they truly are. When two people overflow with love for the other, a very magical relationship gets created. Many soul mate, karmic mate, companion mates, and tantric flame relationships can evolve into a true love experience.

23. *Divine Soul Mate*

When you meet, you will feel a profound sense of coming home, of sharing complementary and compatible life goals. You can be truthful with each other and are able to be your authentic self without the fear of rejection. The lives of divine soul mates are in harmony with each other on a spiritual, mental, emotional, and physical level. Since they have mastered self-love, they raise each other into a higher experience of love. These relationships come together to fulfill spiritual or humanitarian work, and they have many divine timings or destined moments together where their love overflows to help their family or community.

Exercise: Who are your Soul Mates?

This exercise will help you to master more love in your current and past relationships. On a piece of paper, write a list of all the relationships you have experienced. This could include intimate partners as well as family members. Next to each name, decide what type of soul mate experience it was, and then write down the lesson of love you learned from them and what you think you taught them about love. For example:

Tom: Fling—taught me how to be a sexually powerful woman and not to be ashamed of my body. I taught him how to experience easy, unattached love.

Leith: Bad Apple—taught me that I am worth more and that under no circumstances do I deserve to be put down. I taught him that he should not belittle someone in order to receive attention.

The Power of Discernment

At every given moment you have the ability to use discernment. This means that you are able to judge where another person is operating from. This gives you clues as to why the person is interacting with you in certain ways and the quality of love that they are capable of. Discernment is vital to protect your heart and help you navigate through your relationships. It is a gift of your female intuition, and you must learn to use it always.

Once you have assessed a person, you can then adjust what to receive from them and what not to receive from them. This will protect you from having your heart broken or thinking you will get married when the relationship is only ever meant to be a fling. Remember that words, actions, emotions, and thoughts are all vibrations, and you must learn to become aware of the deeper intentions behind everything. Someone can say something nice to you, and at the same time be feeling jealous of you. Or you may notice someone doing a kind act, such as opening a door, but their intentions are not honorable.

When you can discern the intention behind every movement, you will be able to interpret how aligned or not aligned the person is to love. Through this ability you will learn to navigate through people and life with greater clarity.

The key is to stay connected to the great field of love that surrounds you for guidance, and always remain true to the power of love that exists within you. This important connection is available to you at any given time and helps you navigate through your relationships. Remember that you are never alone; you are completely supported by love itself no matter how confused, anxious, or lonely you become in your relationships. Love will be your greatest lover, so keep choosing to fall in love with love itself.

There Are as Many Soul Mates as There Are Stars in the Sky

There are as many different soul mate experiences as there are stars in the sky. No two are alike, and some are capable of journeying with you through many different soul mate dynamics. The more qualities of love you are able to master, the more fluid and easier your relationships will become. The more you are centered in love, the more you will be able to give your partner the skills to center themselves in love. Our ability to pass on love through our words, thoughts, ideas, and actions in every given moment teaches those around us to behave in a more evolved way. The path of love requires that you lead, be patient, and above all, not be tempted to be spiteful, nasty, revengeful, or bitter when you have been hurt. It requires this of your partner, too, if you are to sustain a healthy relationship. If your partner does not choose to step up and experience love with you, then they will naturally remain at a lower vibration while you continue to evolve. Sometimes a breakup is exactly what needs to happen in order to create the space for a new relationship that does vibrate with love.

"Love is not dependent upon another person, but on an eternal source that exists within and around you."

The path of love will bring you soul mates—both those out of alignment and those in alignment with you—so you learn to find your own alignment. Only though this will you understand that love is not dependent upon another person, but on an eternal source that exists within and around you. So treasure all of the soul mate experiences that you have. Whether they are good relationships or bad, they each have occurred to benefit the progression of your soul toward mastering love and loving the self. Through this process, the ultimate quest of becoming your own soul mate and being 'one' with love can be achieved.

Reflection:

1. List all of your relationships and the type of soul mate experiences you have had. What lessons did they teach you?
2. Did any of your relationships cover two or more soul mate categories? Did any keep evolving into a new form?
3. In each relationship that you have had, explore how it helped you to master more love in yourself. In what ways did even the bad relationships teach you how to honor yourself?
4. Which has been your most destructive and damaging relationship? Why? What advice would you give your past self?
5. Why is discernment important in relationships?
6. How does self-love improve your ability to discern the truth of others?
7. Explain what this means to you: "The path of love will bring you soul mates—both those out of alignment and those in alignment with you—so you learn to find your own alignment."
8. Explain what this means to you: "Love is not dependent upon another person, but on an eternal source that exists within and around you."

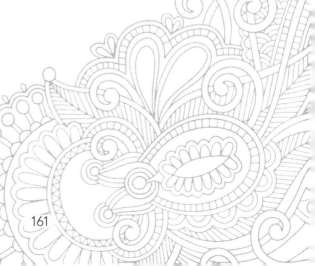

11

The Puzzle Of Love

To exchange love with another person is the sweetest adventure you will ever have. But to master love with another person is a roller coaster that will have you caught in a constant cycle of enlightenment, destruction, and enlightenment again. At times love will make you feel giddy and alive, or so cared for that your self-worth increases. Love can also distract you, making you long and desire. It can create fantasy lands and obsessions that consume you night and day. Sometimes your love can be betrayed, making you wild and filled with revenge. Or you might be dismissed and neglected until you feel your specialness has been forgotten. Every time love breaks, a little part of you will break, too, and you feel as if you are dying inside. These moments can make you feel rejected and unworthy. But over time through the innocence of your heartbreaking, you will learn that love is not an external force; it's an internal one. Every time your hearts breaks, the pain of loneliness will force you to love yourself back to health. It will teach you that you can heal your own heart and nobody in this world can love you as much you can love yourself.

This never-ending game of destruction and rebuilding, plays out so you can transform and expand into a more sublime experience of love with yourself, and a more profound union with others. Every single relationship you have will take you on this journey. In long-term relationships, the cycle of enlightenment to destruction and back to enlightenment, can be played out multiple times where breakups and reunions occur regularly. Sometimes the relationship will force you to choose your own self-worth over the demands of others. Other times it will require you to compromise and honor the needs of your partner first. It's a constant game of readjusting, standing in your truth, and choosing the values of love over your own egoic needs or insecurities. Every situation and every relationship you enter into offers a puzzle of love you need to solve. It is a constant dynamic of reconstruction until both parties feel empowered to exist from their truth. Once you understand that every relationship challenge, hardship, obstacle, or conflict that occurs is really just the universe showing you the areas where you have not mastered love within yourself, the journey into love becomes a beautiful dance.

This puzzle of love forms for many reasons—from the polarization of male and female energy as both parties learn to create balance, to the dynamic play of relationships which include: dismantling expectations, changing yourself to enhance the reflection of love your partner gives you, healing broken love patterns acquired in childhood, and most importantly learning to love yourself more than anyone else can. This game cannot be escaped and will often play out without you even noticing it. Below are five common ways the puzzle of love is played out in relationships:

1. *Dismantling Expectations*

Since there is an innate desire to experience love, people are often caught in an array of romantic illusions as they try to achieve the perfect love story. Subconsciously you are programmed to expect fulfillment from another person as opposed to realizing the fulfilment of love within the self first. This illusion comes from romance novels, television, friends, nursery rhymes, films, magazines, your own family, ballads, songs, poetry, myths, legends, and fairy tales. How often have you fantasied about meeting Prince (Princess) Charming, who rescues you from your troubles and makes all your dreams come true? The unconscious need to fulfill this illusion becomes the driving force that attracts and creates unhealthy relationships.

Such scenarios include:

- Expecting a relationship to cure loneliness
- Feeling it is a partner's responsibility to make you happy
- Thinking that once you are in a relationship, all your problems will be resolved like magic
- The expectation to be financially provided for by your partner—house, car, exotic holidays, handbags, shoes, etc.
- Requiring your partner to look, behave, act, or love in certain ways. This mindset will definitely limit your ability to attract a partner into your life—true love can never be boxed.

2. *History Repeats*

Many patterns that develop in relationships reflect what has been observed in childhood from the way your parents related to each other. Unconsciously you will seek to resolve the broken love they or you experienced by attracting partners with similar personalities to your mother or father. Even though there is no desire to repeat what happened in childhood, history does repeat itself. This is because the patterns of the previous generations have not been resolved, and they need to be so that love can flow freely again into the next generations. Love should flow easily between people without being tangled up in distorted thinking or corrupted actions. Unfortunately, your parents and their parents before and so on have, for various reasons, distorted their understanding of love. Then they projected it onto their spouse to resolve it and vice versa. This play created the family drama that you may have experienced as a child.

It is essential that you become aware of the patterns that exist in your family as well as the patterns that occur in your partner's. Then you must become aware of how they transpire into your relationship with each other. Every partner must take responsibility for his or her issues and choose to transform them. Together through communication you can help each other resolve the broken patterns of love before they create unnecessary drama in your union. You cannot escape your family

165

patterns, but you can choose to heal them so future generations have an easier journey of mastering love.

3. *The Mirror*

Like attracts like; people mirror us in positive and negative ways. The saying "people bring out the best in you, or the worst in you" applies here. Human relationships are designed to help you master love. They become the perfect platform for your soul to be triggered so the distorted beliefs you hold can evolve into wiser, more loving, and more compassionate thoughts.

Subconsciously you will attract partners who mirror your issues so you are confronted by the behaviors you need to shift. Just like a mirror, the reflection will not change until you do. If you do not grow out of limiting patterns, the same type of people, reflecting the same issues, will keep showing up in your life again and again. For example, if you are very emotionally demanding, chances are you will attract a partner with the same needs. You want your needs met, and your partner is unable to meet them because they have exactly the same needs, and they are expecting you to meet theirs. It is a no-win situation unless you fulfill the need within you. The aim of the game is keep transforming the limiting beliefs that keep you from experiencing love. No relationship will grow if both parties hold on to distorted love patterns. Such beliefs could include:

- I must reject my partner before he/she rejects me.
- If I ignore my partner, then he/she will give me more attention.
- Love is painful.
- Love is abusive.
- Love always leaves me.
- I always feel alone in relationships.
- Every time I fall in love I get rejected.
- There was not enough love in my family.
- I am still carrying a heartbreak from a previous relationship.
- Everyone else falls in love except me.
- I am unsure how to receive love.
- I feel unsafe in relationships.

- I am always misunderstood.
- I am afraid of intimacy and affection.

The more you evolve, the more your partner will have the opportunity to evolve because neither of you is locking the other in an unhealthy paradigm. However, if you are in a toxic or abusive relationship, you should not continue trying to fix yourself in order to fix your partner. In these cases, looking into a broken mirror will only give you a broken reflection. You must end the relationship and then heal the limiting beliefs that attracted mistreatment in the first place.

4. Games

So many games are played in the name of love. These games are usually played from patterns of neediness, dependency, possessiveness, jealousy, power, control and domination - all stemming from distorted perceptions of love. Of course, when you play games, your partner will respond by playing games back. No one ever wins—only heart break and entanglement gets created. The corrupted love games that cause unhealthy relationships can include:

- *Withholding*: This is where one partner withholds love and affection in order to hurt or get their way.
- *Projecting*: When one transfers their issues and beliefs onto their partner without considering their partner's truth.
- *Complaining*: This is unnecessarily expressing dissatisfaction without actively trying to provide a solution.
- *Manipulating*: Coercing and influencing your partner to do as you desire.
- *Gaslighting*: This occurs when one partner lies and psychologically manipulates the other to doubt their own sanity.
- *Threatening*: Occurs when one partner maintains their power by causing the other to feel vulnerable or at risk.
- *Ultimatums*: Demanding certain terms from one's partner, in which the rejection of those terms will result in a breakdown of relationship.
- *Ignoring*: This is when one partner intentionally refuses to acknowledge or take notice of the other.

- *Blaming:* Similar to complaining, blaming is constantly declaring that your partner is at fault or wrong without offering a constructive solution.
- *Punishing:* This occurs when one partner inflicts the other with an emotional, physical or monetary penalty as retribution for a perceived offence.
- *Diminishing:* When one partner makes the other feel invaluable or worthless.
- *Possessiveness:* This occurs when one partner wants to own and control how the other thinks, feels, dresses and what they can and can't do etc.
- *Stonewalling:* When one partner refuses to communicate and express emotions.

The reason relationships get caught in the destructive loop of playing games is complex. Usually it indicates healing is required for the relationship to evolve. When you are after the experience of true love, you cannot play games that get you lost in a labyrinth of unfulfillment. Often this will require you to lead by example until your partner discovers a new way to relate. This is where you develop excellent communications skills; you are able to listen, learn to maturely confront issues without fighting or becoming defensive, apply the virtues of love, and be willing to guide yourself and your partner to heal so you both can continuously become the better versions of yourselves.

5. *Sexual Trauma and Sexual Shadow*

Everything in this universe is moving towards love. All the sexual experiences you agreed to encounter were attempts to experience love. Unfortunately, due to the selfish or uneducated behavior of others or a disempowered sense of self, many sexual experiences may have been far removed from the experience of love, often leaving memories that scar the psyche and distort the emotions. In order to experience your sexuality as a sacred experience, you must heal the subconscious split between love and sex, as well as the separation of spirituality and sexuality. Then and only then can your love sacredly and intimately unite with the love of another on a physical, sexual, emotional, mental, and spiritual level. This is the experience of true union.

Example of experiences that split love from sex:

- Being touched in a way that is not been an expression of love
- Giving in when your soul and body say no
- Not having your boundaries respected
- Feeling obliged to pleasure another
- Feeling guilty for experiencing pleasure
- Feeling shameful, dirty, embarrassed about your body, your sexuality, and about your desires
- Being made to feel shameful or embarrassed about your body and sexuality by someone else

Examples of experiences of love uniting with sex:

- Being touched with love
- Having your boundaries honored and your requests met with care
- Fusing heart and sexual energy together to nourish the other
- Harnessing sexual energy to access the truth of yourself and your partner
- Experiencing an intimate exchange of love through physical contact
- Giving and receiving bliss, joy, and freedom

Sometimes the body shuts down in fear and shock as a form of defense when it has encountered something other than love. This could be experienced as closing, contracting, shutting down, numbness, pain, discomfort, checking out, not being able to relax, thinking too much during sex, body shame, insecurities, or having a feeling that something is wrong with you. Shadows are formed within the psyche, creating grief, sadness, or anger. These become locked memories and trapped emotions. Applying the healing process in chapter Eight—*The Lotus Transcends from Her Mud*—will help you heal your sexual shadow experiences.

Dismantling the shadows within is a transformative process as you finally stop running away, pushing, or denying what is hidden. This frees your energy so you can accept, hold, liberate, and love all the broken parts until you feel whole again. An incredible amount of wisdom and compassion emerges from this process, which ultimately translates as a greater capacity to love both yourself and others.

Just like a vase that has broken into many pieces and has shattered on the floor, you have to look at each piece, examine what happened to it, and figure out how it fits back into the vase. The vase represents you. You then glue these pieces back together with love. You love yourself whole again.

Please note: if you've experienced abuse, rape, or molestation, and you feel recovery still needs to take place, I highly recommend finding someone who is skilled and qualified to support you.

6. Male and Female Energy

In this human experience, love becomes polarized between masculine and feminine qualities that ultimately complement and support each other to unite into oneness. Every person has both masculine and feminine qualities, and we tend to seek partners who synergistically complete what we lack and vice versa.

Feminine and masculine energies are constantly dancing within to create wholeness, and in turn dancing with others to create balance. Masculine energy is all about consciousness, knowledge, wisdom, and logic. Practical in its efforts, the masculine aspect provides structure, discipline, safety, and security for the feminine energies to birth ideas and create beauty.

Masculine energy provides focus, intention, vision, and wisdom to help build those ideas, whereas feminine energy desires to create harmony and dream heaven into existence. In order to feel secure enough to grow, feminine energies need the protection of masculine energies. Then feminine energy will nurture and encourage masculine energy to lead her creations into existence. This grants the masculine energy a sense of power and pride because the feminine has given him purpose, and so he chooses to care and nurture for her even more. The feminine feels more secure in being loved and so generates love to create beauty, peace, and harmony in the relationship. Each learns from the other and then surrenders to the appropriate leader so their desires of true love are manifested in physical reality. This partnership can happen internally on an emotional level through communication or externally in practical and physical ways such as creating a business. Each partner supplies what the other is missing or has the skills to substitute what the other lacks. Through this dynamic match, each partner has the keys to unlock their partner's greatness, which would otherwise stay dormant. Through this process they elevate each other to relate in more loving and mature ways.

On the other hand, if the masculine energy behaves in immature ways, it can criticize, dominate, and become possessive of the feminine energy. This will make the female energy collapse into feeling rejected and trapped, making her become self-obsessive, unworthy, neurotic, or desperately seeking validation and approval. When the female energy gets stuck in being a victim, her power to create is lost. Instead she gains position through manipulation or by being overly caring or responsible or superficially friendly to be noticed and get attention. The male energy can take advantage of this and drain the female energy for his own egoic needs. Instead of protecting and encouraging the female energy to blossom, the masculine energy will use the female energy to serve him. This can further make him more dominating, possessive, and critical, and continues the cycle of collapsing the female energy.

This energy polarization of masculine and feminine energies either creates a positive tension that generates the magnetic energy needed to create union, or it generates a negative tension that creates destruction. But both partners, regardless of gender, will isolate between taking the feminine or masculine lead, depending on the dynamics that the circumstance creates.

Since we all have masculine and feminine energies, this dance also happens within so that we learn to support our own growth and maturity. As our internal masculine and feminine energies learn to love each other, there is an equal desire for our external energy to help and love other people. Through this longing, we invite other souls to dance with us.

The purpose of a relationship is not to have someone else complete you, but rather to share your completeness with them. In order to obtain this, the puzzles of love will continuously play out in your life and never end, no matter how evolved you become. This is because the experience of enlightenment is infinite, and this creates infinite situations in the physical world to master love. You therefore will keep attracting soul mates in all forms to play out the game of love so that you keep evolving. They will come in all shapes and sizes. Some will repulse you and others will enliven you, but all will hold a key that unlocks a deeper awareness.

Returning Your Relationship Back to Love

The puzzle of love between people creates a dynamic dance that can make us feel elated, deflated, and sometimes both at once. It is never easy because the paradox between two people is completely unique. In fact, never before and never again will the same combination of two people exist. Since the combination of every partnership only ever happens once in the universe, the methods you use to elevate each other into a more profound experience of love is completely unique. That's why there is never one magic formula that will solve all your relationships. There are, however, four keys that you always have available to return your relationship back to love.

1. Communication

The greatest key to a successful relationship is being able to communicate your wants, needs, and desires in an articulate and loving way. Many of us have not been taught how to be kind with words. Words are powerful and can either bless or curse someone. You must learn to choose the words that both educate your partner and help them to understand your truth. Communication also involves being able to listen to your partner and requires that you are able to hear all that they say—not just what you want to hear. A good listener is also able to hear beyond their partner's words and hear what they don't say or are unable to say. As you develop good communication with your partner, you will indirectly master authentic relating. You should aim for a relationship dynamic that allows both parties to create so much trust and support that only the authentic truth of the other can be accepted and honored.

2. Letting the Other Person Be Who They Are

One of the hardest things to do in a relationship is to let the other person be who they truly are. Without being aware, you may project onto them who you want them to be or obligate them to behave in a certain way. This occurs because you have subconscious beliefs that force you to believe that relationships can only function in a certain way. These limiting beliefs about relationships come from our parents, society, and past relationships. Such beliefs lock both parties into living a life that does not fully resonate with their authentic truth. An evolved relationship, however, allows each partner to be who they truly are. Love comes from freedom, and so you must give your partner the freedom to express their truth. Maybe one partner wants to go on vacation by themselves; maybe the other partner needs to dye their hair green to feel alive and empowered. Whatever their truth is, it is important to express and find ways to grant your partner the freedom to experience it. Life is always changing, relationships are always growing, and freedom allows love to exist through it all. The more you allow your partner to be free to live their truth, the more they will allow you to live yours. Likewise, the more you allow your partner to live their truth, the more you will be able to let yourself live more of your truth. Through this process you allow both yourself and your partner to blossom into a more exquisite version of yourselves.

3. Tactile Affection

Cuddles, kisses, touching, hugs, and eye gazing are beautiful expressions of love and can reset the dynamics of a relationship. This is because tactile affection does not require words to communicate love and helps to release love hormones that calm the nervous system. If you have been arguing or fighting or are lost for the right words, then tactile displays of affection are an excellent remedy to return both partners to love so resolution can take place. Making time to be affectionate for at least thirty minutes a day will increase both parties' ability to be more compatible with each other. There will be more kindness, more care with words, and often cuddles can lead to more passionate activities. If it is a little awkward or scary to be completely present without being able to use words, begin by setting a timer for five minutes, ten minutes, fifteen minutes, and so on. You could dedicate the time to just kissing or touching or eye gazing. When you both get comfortable, you can try the freedom of flowing from one form of affection to the next.

4. Reflection

This is probably your most needed key; it's required in every relationship dynamic, especially the relationship you have with yourself. Reflection allows you to pause and take time to assess the true dynamics being played out. You'll be able to work out if it's your stuff you are projecting into the relationship, or your partner's stuff. Or, perhaps it's some old hurt that has surfaced to be healed, so you can step back into your power. Maybe you need some space to reorganize who you are after a period of personal growth, and what you are now needing from the relationship. Just as we all need time out to meditate and create stillness within, taking time out to reflect will offer the guidance you require to navigate your relationship back to the peace of love. Remember, as a sensually enlightened woman, you have all the keys to master yourself, so always begin there.

Dealing with Heartbreak

On the journey into love, you won't be able to escape the experience of a broken heart. There are thousands of ways your heart can break—a relationship breakup, being shouting at as a child, someone dear to you dying, or your own unworthiness or self-hatred. Sometimes your heart will break a little, and other times it will break a lot. But every time your heart breaks, it smashes through an illusion that can no longer be maintained, a fantasy that cannot be made real, an unfair projection, the realization that what you took for granted is no longer there, or simply just how much you really loved someone.

I remember my first heartbreak; it was the most devastating experience. I came home from visiting my family in Australia, and my then-boyfriend (now husband) asked for a us to have a break in our relationship. As soon as he told me, I felt as though he ripped out my heart and sliced it in two. My whole life, including the future I had planned, got swallowed up, and I felt completely empty without him. I begged him to not leave me, I didn't sleep, and I couldn't eat for days. To his credit, during the break, he did come over to my house and forced me to eat. Still, for me, it was as if I experienced death.

Once, I had gotten over the shock, the anger, revenge, and all the reasons why he should stay with me, I made the decision that I had to love myself more than the love he gave to me. Every day I would sit in meditation and welcome, all the love that poured out of my heart for him, to come back to me. Eventually the hole in my heart was filled with self-love, and I rose out of the pain.

After two months of being apart, my boyfriend realised that I was the one for him. He invited me to spend New Year's with him so we could reconcile. By that time, I had recovered and had become so strong in being my own soul mate that I remembered thinking, *"Oh, I already made plans for New Year's"*, and was disappointed that he was disrupting them. I healed my heart so thoroughly, I actually became so secure and independent, I no longer needed him to feel whole. This raised me to a new experience of love, one where I had so much love for myself that it overflowed to gift him with a new experience of love. Through the process of breaking up, we returned to the relationship wiser, more mature, more respectful, and much more aware of how to allow each other to exist in our own truth. The night we reunited was magic, our lovemaking so deeply loving and caring. We were able to give more to each other, instead of our previous dynamic of needing and expecting.

Heartbreaks are inevitable, and they will happen even in long-term relationships as each person chooses to return back to their truth. The reality is that on a very deep level, no one is actually compatible; each person in their authenticity is profoundly unique. This becomes more and more apparent as you blossom into your truth. As a society we spend more time trying to fit in than actually learning to be our true selves. Your closest relationships will force you to become yourself, they will push your buttons and trigger you in unexpected ways. Every relationship teaches you how to master love in a very unique way and so teaches you how to master yourself. It is only when you master yourself that you will learn to navigate through all your relationships with greater precision. You will know when to act, when to stop, when to say yes, and when to say no. As you master the virtues of love within yourself, you will also master the virtues of love with your partners.

This leads me to the second break my husband and I had in our relationship. It was about three years after the birth of my daughter, and I had taken myself deep into the path of sensual enlightenment. I had learned to become my own soul mate, and I cultivated my sexual energy to unite with my heart, so I could always be in love. I learned to become empowered and full of the self-worth needed to generate my own source of abundance. As I grew into myself, I become more resentful of my partner who was not growing along the path that I projected for 'me'. I began to reject him for not being good enough, and he reciprocated by rejecting me. This cycle continued for months until eventually there was a wall of silent resentment and unhappiness between us.

Eventually, we reached a point where we needed to end the relationship; we did not end our relationship in a bitter way, we just knew it was unhealthy to continue. I moved out and it was the best thing that could have happened—the months of silent resentment collapsed; the blame and rejection ended. There was forgiveness, freedom, and finally peace. Within a few weeks of being 'single', I felt a pull of energy desiring to connect back with him. We went on some dates. We laughed, we kissed, we made love, and before I knew it, we were back together in a completely new relationship. There was a new chemistry, a new spark of new love that willed us to keep connecting. We returned back to the purity of love that had always existed between us. We were teenagers in love again, but we had needed to completely let go of our old dynamic first. Heartbreaks—although painful—can be completely renewing for yourself and your relationships.

Here is my ultimate heartbreak remedy—it can be used to heal your broken heart or just to return back to your truth if the relationship has caused you to wobble. (You can find the recorded version in my FREE *Rebirth Into Love* Online course. Go to www.vanyasilverten.com to locate it.)

Heartbreak Remedy

1. Begin in a meditation position. Place your hands on your heart and breathe deeply until you feel more present in your body.
2. When you are ready, visualize all the love that flows from your heart toward your partner coming back to you. You can use your hands to call your love back to you. On an inhale, breathe your energy back into your heart. Sadness or anger may begin to come up. If it does, just exhale it out and inhale your love back in. Eventually through this process, you will have a feeling of returning back to yourself.
3. Now visualize yourself surrounded by love itself. Place your hands on your knees, and as you inhale, visualize breathing love into your heart. Exhale, continuing to let go of the sadness or anger in your heart. Repeat this until your heart feels full of love

and you remember that you come from love and are surrounded by love.

4.   Place one hand on your heart and one hand on your womb space. Inhale your sexual energy up to your heart, and then exhale it through your heart center. Repeat this process until you feel your sexual energy filling you up and completing your heart. This may bring tears to your eyes as you supply yourself with what you partner previously did. Eventually you will smile with joy for being able to fulfill and make yourself whole again.

Always remember that every heartbreak you experience is a blessing in disguise—it will force you to return back to your truth. It will make you stronger in yourself, wiser in love, and more empowered to transform your relationships. Although they are never pleasant, the recovery of each heartbreak will become easier and easier, until you embrace them as a cathartic up-leveling into a more sublime experience of love.

Reflection:

1. Describe what this means to you: "The purpose of a relationship is not to have someone else complete you, but rather to share your completeness with them."
2. List all the things you expect from your partner, and in doing so, notice the barriers they form that stop love from flowing.
3. What distorted family love patterns have transpired into your relationships?
4. What distorted love patterns from your partner's family have affected your relationship?
5. In what ways does your partner mirror your positive and negative qualities?
6. What unhealthy games do you play in order to receive love?
7. Where has love split from your intimate experiences?
8. Do you find it easier to play the masculine or feminine role? How does this dynamic play out in yourself and in relationships?
9. Explore the ways to return your relationship to love — communication, letting your partner be who they are, tactile affection, reflection, and so on. Which is the easiest? Which is the hardest? Why?
10. Explore all the heartbreaks you have experienced in your life or in your current/last relationship. Sum up what they have taught you.

12

The Union of Sensual Enlightenment

Your path of sensual enlightenment has taught you how to love yourself so much that your unique truth and your inner beauty have become your outer radiance. Through each chapter you have learned to become intimate with yourself, so you can become more intimate with life. Intimacy is the ability to get closer to your truth, be present with your wounds, accept everything that makes you *you*, keep choosing to open and reveal more and more of your beauty, and be free to discover what you don't know about yourself as well. The intimacy you learn to have with yourself will teach you how to honor yourself, be independent, trust yourself and therefore others, and most importantly, it will ensure that you love and care for yourself immensely. The intimacy you have with yourself will become the intimacy you learn to have with another. Just as you have journeyed to fall in love with loving yourself into love, you will long to fall in love with someone else so you can both experience falling in love with love together. True intimacy occurs when there is self-awareness, and a trust in the mechanics and dynamics of how love plays out. True intimacy requires both partners to share their essence, their self- love, their life wisdom and their sexual energy to awaken their partner.

Intimacy is the exchange of affection with touch, cuddles, kissing, and sexual connection. It can also include conversations, eye gazing, and a general sharing of all aspects of life. The love exchange can be profound and orgasmic in all of these situations. Saying the right words to your partner can open them up to receive the love that flows from you to them. A gentle touch on a sensitive part of the body can unlock your partner's beauty. Looking into each other's eyes, kissing, or giving a compliment can awaken an orgasmic response. Just as you have learned that your sexual energy is magnetized to the love within you, likewise your sexual energy is magnetized to the love inside your partner and vice versa. This exchange creates a charge of attraction that often feels electric. At other times it may feel as if the other person is filling you with their energy, giving the sensation that they are completing you or replenishing you. In some cases you may even feel as if your partner's energy has "found" parts of you that you never knew existed. This can make you feel so ignited that you suddenly feel empowered to express more of your truth.

I put this into practice with my husband by requesting that his love and sexual energy should ignite me in ways other than intercourse. As I opened myself to receive, through his kisses I orgasmed, through him touching my ears and hair, I orgasmed, through him looking at me with so much care I orgasmed, and even once when he gave me a compliment, I orgasmed because I could feel the electric love he transferred through his body into me. Our bodies are designed to give and receive love in subtle and orgasmic ways.

> **'Your sexual energy is magnetized to the**
> **love that is within your partner.'**

As both partners choose to get closer and share more of their energy, their auric fields unite, creating a sensation of being one with each other. You may begin to feel what your partner is thinking or feeling. You will begin to make choices for your life that benefit both of you. You will begin to feel as though you belong to each other, offering the protection and security that a family provides. This is a double- sided coin. On one side, becoming familiar with your partner can lead you to believe you know what's best for them, then you might over step boundaries, and begin to choose their life for them. This will bypass their individuality and put a halt to the process of experiencing true love. The other side of the coin is that the more you are able to merge your body, mind, heart, spirit, and sexuality with your partner, the more you have the opportunity to melt and disappear into love with them. Your intimate exchanges will feel as if your uniqueness is disappearing, and that your connection unifies to the point, where both of you become the great field of love. From this place, energy is exchanged between your atoms and molecules, and your souls merge on a deep level. Finally, the missing information needed to return to love is given. These profoundly intimate moments will make you feel full of love, and your perception of reality will never be the same again. Your vibration will increase and expand because it has received, given, generated, and reunited back to love.

'Consent and intimacy go hand in hand.'

Consent and intimacy go hand in hand; one cannot exist without the other. In order to open yourself and get more connected with you partner, you must choose to. And in order for your partner to get more connected to you, he or she also must choose to. Consent gives you the freedom and power to make choices for your body and your life. It is the knowing that you have complete sovereignty over every aspect of your body and that you are never obligated to submit to the needs of another.

Consent is not a one-time event when you first meet, or something that is transferable to the next intimate moment. Consent is something that happens every moment in a relationship when a new situation or dynamic arises, and it can be withdrawn at any time. Just because you have been intimate with someone in the past, does not mean you have to be intimate with them again. This also applies to long-term relationships. Just because you have consented to intimacy a hundred times before, it does not mean you have to consent today or tomorrow. It could mean that you choose to be intimate next week. You can choose to kiss someone but not be sexually intimate with them; you can choose to cuddle without kissing; you can choose to touch without talking. Consent creates boundaries and parameters of how the intimate union between two people is experienced. And each encounter, when honored, can be orgasmically beautiful if you accept the dynamic and choose to experience the unique love that comes from it.

The key to consent is honor the other person's boundaries by adhering to their requests. The best requests come in the form of direct and clear communication of what your wants, needs, and boundaries are. However, you can softly communicate what you are willing to consent to through your body language, such as turning away from your partner, brushing off their advances, or redirecting the way they interact with you. In situations where your partner is not registering and honoring your requests, you have the right to loudly say no, push them away, or stand up and leave the situation. You have many consent options, and the more you let go of your shyness, unworthiness, and submissive patterns, the easier it will be to display your boundaries with you voice, your eyes, your body language, and your energy field. A "no" can come in many forms, and each one is a powerful tool that ensures your sovereignty.

The beauty of the path into sensual enlightenment is that you create a strong presence with your sexual energy and a sense of empowerment with self-love. Both are essential ingredients that help you understand the standard of care and intimacy you require. To be definite about what you are willing to accept and experience in any given moment is power. This will later translate into the ability to make clearer decisions in business or give more direct instructions to help manifest your visions into reality. On a fundamental level you learn consent first with yourself because you must choose what is right for you. Next you learn to communicate your needs and desires to another person, and later you are able to command and influence the life around you. When you choose to stand in your power and express your truth, life has no choice but to reflect your brilliance. Your ability to master consent also helps you to master your life. Your ability to honor your partner's boundaries and consent wishes helps your partner to master their life as well. Every boundary, every request you make, is an opportunity to navigate your relationship toward love. Consent is not just about saying no; it is also about guiding your partner to interact with your truth.

'Consent guides your partner to interact with your truth.'

Consent is extremely important in all intimate, romantic, and sexual relationships. This is because sexual energy is the primary force that creates the magnetism for two souls to come together in union. However, if partners are unable to process their sexual energy through the energy of love, the untamed nature of the sexual energy can create situations you may find unsafe. Such situations could include being pressured or forced to do something you do not like, which in extreme cases could lead to rape, or your partner might put their needs over yours, making you feel that they are taking advantage of you. Sexual energy in its raw state can be very arousing, but if you want to navigate your relationship to love, then consent and communication are vital.

Communicating your intimate needs takes courage and commitment, and it takes a lot of understanding to discover your partner's needs and desires as well. Clear and sometimes unedited or diplomatic communication makes it possible to work through any blocks that limit your capacity to fully enjoy sexual pleasure and the experience of physical intimacy. This ability is really a very refined version of consent, something that relationships naturally grow into if there is a lot of mutual respect.

When both partners articulate what is intimately satisfying in an open space of trust, freedom is created to explore each other. Entering into the depths of your partner's landscape of love is very exciting. As you both reveal yourself, you eventually create a lovemaking culture that is unique to your union. Cultivating the art of love is just like cultivating any other art form. It comes with patience, practice, and time. Patience—to both communicate and understand the blocks and needs of your partner and yourself. Practice—to refine the skills that open the other to experience more love. Time—to slow down and open to the presence of each other. Lovemaking is not fast food. With patience, practice, and time, much healing and transformation can take place during intimate union.

Each time you and your partner honor each other, more trust will develop. Trust is the most important ingredient in a relationship because it allows you to feel safe enough to keep revealing your essence. Your essence is the most magical part of you—it is your unique vibration of love, and it desires to shine from your cells and unite to your partner's essence. And your partner's unique essence desires to shine from his or her cells into you. Each person assists the other to return to their purity, so more love can flow and create union.

This is why when you leave each other, even if it's just for a work trip, you will often feel your body longing for your partner to return because you have become one with them. This experience gives rise to the expression "I have found the one" or "he is a part of me." Such a merging can take place with any couple that chooses to meet each other with love. You can have this true love experience for one minute with someone who is merely a fling, or you can experience it for years with a long-term mate. True love is never bound to one person, although it does require that you be completely present with the virtues of love for the time that you are in exchange. But the exchange of love goes beyond the paradigm of you and your partner; it is ultimately an exchange with the love that exists through the divine universe.

'True love is ultimately an exchange with the great field of love.'

When consent, communication, trust, and respect become the foundation of a relationship, the sexual energy of both people are elevated into a more loving state. The sexual energy then sublimates from the primary need to be satisfied to a more elevated desire of awakening, fulfilling, and even healing their partner so they can experience more love. Just as you have discovered that your own sexual energy is magnetized to the love within you, your partner's sexual energy is also magnetized to the love within you and vice versa. Your partner's sexual energy has the potential to ignite the love that exists in your arms, legs, toes, fingers, sexual palace, breasts, ears, eyes, and every cell in your body. This is why that after lovemaking, you will feel radiant and beautiful. Your partner has used their sexual energy to cause your unique essence to blossom and radiate out of your body. This also can occur without intercourse, because sexual energy has the freedom to move anywhere in your body and then into your partner's body. For example, when your sexual energy is directed through your heart chakra toward your partner, it pushes out the vibration of love within you to fill them.

A couple who has learned to sublimate their sexual energy, has the potential to give the love that exists within every cell of their body, to awaken every cell in the other's body, and vice versa. In this way both partners learn to loop together and unite. This then allows them to exchange the super highway of soul information. Each partner gifts the other with their unique essence, which is filled with learnings, awareness, and healing energy needed to elevate the other. This exquisite exchange can take place anywhere at any time. It could occur in the supermarket while choosing fruit, through intentional touching or eye gazing, when being very present with each other during lovemaking, or while having a telephone conversation when both parties are in two different countries. Your sexual energy can travel to unite with the love that exists within your partner—it is not bound to time, space, distance, or direction. This magnetic pull and dynamic exchange can even occur multidimensionally with cosmic mates such as the sun or the stars.

Just before I entered into a long-term relationship with my husband, I had a love affair with the sun. It was an unusually hot summer in London, and I had moved into a flat where the morning sun would come through my bedroom window and greet me every morning. I would take long walks in the parks and the sun would always find me - warming my head, shinning on my arms, touching my cheeks. Our exchange heightened until I felt the sun making love to me daily. Now the sun is very yang (masculine) in nature, and every time the sun would shine its light into me, I felt the parts of me which had be broken by men in past relationships heal. It was as if the sun was recoding me with experience of being loved by divine male love. It was the missing information I needed for a healthy relationship. Towards the end of my love affair with the sun, I joked to 'him' that 'he' never kisses my hand. The next day while at work, two random men kissed my hand, which had never happened before or again since. A month after my love affair with the sun had finished, I began my love affair with the man who was to become my husband.

A sensually enlightened woman is one that can be in a loving exchange with existence. The information received from such exchanges brings the awareness and experience necessary to awaken her to the next level of self-mastery. This is where the virtues of love become an embodiment and a physical experience with another. This is the joy, the laughter, the electrifying touches, the romantic walks where everything feels perfect, and the desire to know each other more that brings deep and meaningful conversations. To embody the virtues of love with your partner will make you friends, lovers, caring companions, and adventurers all at once. You and your partner will help birth the vibration of love through your bodies, the awareness of love through your minds, the harmony of love through your hearts to bless each other, and then the life around you. Together you allow more love to exist in the human experience—from your families to your communities to the environment.

'The virtues of love become an embodiment with your partner.'

The next time you are intimate with your partner, allow yourself to expand and be intimate with the vibration of love that surrounds you both. You will begin to understand that true love does not actually come from one person. Instead you will recognize that the love you have for your partner, is the catalyst to connect you to more love in the universe. In this awareness, you will never feel depleted if you separate from your partner. This is because you have learned your partner is just a vessel, to bring the physical experience of love, for a moment in time. In other words, love itself is choosing to love you through your partner, and likewise love itself is choosing to love your partner through you.

Orgasmic Gifts

As you deepen your experience of intimacy with your partner, and both of you learn to master the vibration of love through each other's bodies, something very beautiful begins to take place. The intimate exchange that you have creates an information highway where you gift each other with the keys to unlock and raise each other's consciousness to your next understanding of love. This occurs because your sexual energy has a highly aroused need to expand and meet the love in your partner and vice versa. In other words, your sexual energy will begin to flow out of your body, taking your essence with it and entering your partner's body as a gift. Your essence is coded with your unique blueprint, which is formed by your consciousness and your spiritual learnings. In this moment you can transfer all of your knowings to your partner so they can evolve and transcend their limitations with your information and vice versa. The universe has an uncanny way of matching you with soul mates who carry the particular information you need to advance your awakenings. This can happen in small ways, such as gaining a new understanding of how to relate to self-love, or it can occur in a more physical way, when your partner's essence provides new fuel to rejuvenate your body. This is why you may feel more radiant and beautiful in the presence of certain people or after lovemaking. When your body is energized with your partner's sexual energy, your orgasmic potential begins to heighten with greater intensity.

'You can learn to ride the orgasmic energy
that emits from your partner's body.'

If we take this understanding to the next level, you can actually learn to ride the orgasmic energy that emits from your partner's body. The easiest way to do this is to notice where your partner's sexual energy is emitting. Perhaps it is around their genitals or from their hands, heart, or erogenous zones. You may feel it as warmth, heat, fire, electricity, sparkly energy, or an arousing sensation that radiates from a particular body part. Welcome their sexual energy into your body; breathe their sexual energy into the cells of your body and let it activate the vibration of love that exists inside of you. As this occurs, you may notice the parts of your body that are stimulated by their sexual energy beginning to orgasm. If you welcome your partner's sexual energy into the erogenous zones of your ears, for example, you may feel your ears sparkling with delight. If you welcome their sexual energy into your breasts, you may notice your breasts awakening and your nipples becoming erect. You may welcome their sexual energy into your vagina and womb space, and without any physical penetration, your entire sexual palace can orgasm because you have been penetrated energetically by your lover. As you orgasm, your partner can then learn to channel the orgasmic energy that emits from your body back into their body to orgasm. This gives both of you the potential to ride each other's orgasmic waves without touch, penetration, or kissing. If both of you can master this connection, then when you do begin to have physical contact, the orgasmic potential can be mind- and body-blowing. You can also practice this exchange at a distance from each other. Or take this experience to the next level by inviting the great field of love to flow through each of your bodies, thus intensifying the orgasmic exchange. This will give you the sensation of being made love to simultaneously by both your partner and the universe—a truly ecstatic and profoundly fulfilling experience that will leave you feeling whole and complete. (To remember the potential of your orgasmic experience, please reread chapter four, "Riding the Orgasmic Waves of Love.")

Exercise: How to Ignite Your Partner with Love from the Universe - *refer to figure 12:*

1. Begin facing each other in a position that is most comfortable to you both.
2. Spend some time moving through the different intimate exchanges, being present with each one until it generates feelings

of love and deeper connection. You might want to set a timer, and then every five minutes change the way you are relating. You could begin with eye gazing, touching, kissing, or cuddling. Notice how the magnetic charge builds between you both.

3. Next, sit in stillness and be completely present with each other. Notice how your energy is still being exchanged.

4. With intention, both partners guide their sexual energy up to their heart chakra on an inhale, and then exhale it through their chest into their partner's body. To help pump the sexual energy through your body, squeeze your intimate muscles on the inhale and release them on the exhale. Practice this a few times. Then practice reversing it so that on the inhale, you breathe your partner's energy through your heart chakra and exhale it down to your sexual palace. As you do this, you will notice your body becoming energized by your partner. You may even notice love bursting from your cells, creating orgasmic sensations.

5. When you are ready, alternate your breathing so that when you exhale your energy into your partner, your partner consciously inhales it back into their body. During this sequence, you inhale your sexual energy up to your heart and then exhale it into your partner. As you do, intend and visualize the love within you shining into your partner. Your partner would then, on an inhale, receive your energy into their body and direct it down to their sexual palace. On the exhale they direct it from their sexual palace to your sexual palace. Then you would repeat this process, letting the energy build between you. Next you can swap roles so you inhale your partner's energy. Keep doing this until you feel so connected that your individual identity disappears.

6. You can expand this same practice by looping the energy through the chakras from the base to the crown. Or do the same practice focusing on each erogenous zone in the body.

7. When you feel completely merged with you partner and your energy is glowing with their energy, tune into the great field of love that surrounds you both. On an inhale intend that the great field of love enters through your partner's body into your body. Exhale and breathe that love down to your sexual palace and transfer it back to your partner's body. Notice the blissful sensations that blossom through your body—and smile every time you experience them.

8. You can alternate who inhales and exhales, and you can practice breathing the great field of love through different parts of the body. The key is noticing the exchange of energy that is happening between your partner, the great field of love, and you. Notice the different orgasmic reactions that are happening in your body, between you and your partner's body, and between you and the great field of love.

9. End the session by hugging and embracing each other. Then physically disconnect from your partner, each spends a moment being present with the connection you have to the love that surrounds you. If you like, you can inhale love through all of your cells, and then on the exhale, breathe that love down to your sexual palace. Inhale the energy from your sexual palace up to your heart and—if you can—to all of your cells, and then exhale and breathe that beautiful energy through your body, giving it back to the universe. Practice this a few times.

10. Finally, lie down together and spend ten minutes resting, watching, and experiencing your body glowing and exchanging with the divine universe and each other.

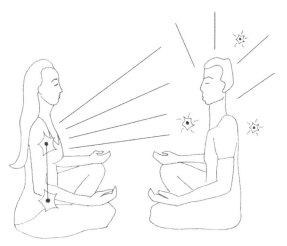

Figure 12: Igniting Your Partner With Universal Love

Once you recognize that every soul mate and intimate experience is an opportunity for you to meet love itself, you will be able to fully recognize that you can have a dynamic love affair with life itself. After all, love is your ultimate soul mate, and since you live in a human body, the life around you becomes the perfect platform for this to play out.

A Dynamic Love Affair with Life

Love affairs are not limited to only one other person; it extends to include every person you meet, every situation you encounter, every cloud that passes, every star that twinkles, and every blade of grass that grows—it is a love affair with life. When your being opens with love for life, your energy flows through your energy pathways, and extends beyond your body to meet the love outside of you and be nourished by it. These energy pathways become your sensual antennas that provide delightful sensory feedback in the form of smells, sounds, visions, and experiences. Anything that does not relay love will be overlooked for something that does, and this is how you are consciously able to enter in the dimension of heaven on earth again and again until it becomes your normal reality. This universe is made up of different vibrationary realities—all you have to do is tune your being like you tune your radio to a particular station.

When you fall in love with life, colors become more vibrant, sounds more intricate, and scents more fragrant. The bubbles in your champagne fizz more, and the simplest daily routines, such as washing your hair, become more luxurious. You will notice every living thing glowing with divine awareness. Just like a bee that becomes intoxicated by the perfume of a flower, your entire female body temple will long for a life that aligns with the delights of love. Every time your heart opens with compassion for another living thing, you help birth the divine universe into life. Through this the energy of love exchanges between you and that which you focus on, your unique vibrations swap and educate the other with missing information. Your souls learn from each other, and an elevation in consciousness occurs. You both rise in love. This could occur in a moment or last for minutes to a lifetime.

Whether this moment is shared with a flower, a person, an animal, or the sun, it is the moment where you fall in love with life. You become aware that the beauty that you desire to experience is actually available to you everywhere and at every moment in the physical world. You simply have to open your being and invite love to enter every aspect of you and your life. You allow the divine consciousness of love to make love to you in as many ways as it can—through songs, messages, conversations, meetings, opportunities, the sunlight on your skin. Every inch of you, from your internal to your external world, deserves to be loved by life. All you have to do is learn to receive it—not an easy task if you have been programmed to give and serve. Just as you need to inhale as much as you need to exhale, you need to learn to receive as much as you need to give. How else will you be able to accept and experience the abundance of love showing up in your life? When you receive, gratitude naturally follows, and this further opens your heart to receive more.

No aspect of love can be secluded or denied, because everything comes from love, everything is evolving toward love, and everything is a gateway to experience more love. Your journey into sensual enlightenment is a never-ending blossoming that will refine you, your relationships and your everyday life with love. These three ways of getting closer to love actually happen simultaneously all the time. You just have to keep transcending the mud within that inhibits this process. The more you love yourself, the more you will able to give love to the right people and the more you learn to open and receive the love life offers you. This is how love flows; it is never limited to one person or one experience—it is a constant continuation. There may be a few bumps, a few challenges, and a few heartbreaks along the way, but each one will teach you how to refine your relationship to love. This is so you can experience a more sublime version of it. Just like winning a game of chess, different situations require you to use different combinations of the virtues of love, so you can move to the next level. Each obstacle and challenge, you face and overcome in your life, strengthens your core to become unshakable with love. To be unshakable with love means that nothing can destroy or diminish your sense of self, because the dynamic power of love resides at your core.

'*To be unshakeable with love means that nothing can destroy or diminish your sense of self.*'

An example is giving birth to a child but experiencing complications that inhibit your desire for a natural birth, which happened to me (as I shared in the introduction). Once I got over the heartbreak of not being able to give birth to my daughter naturally, I made a decision that her birth would be as magical as a natural birth. I opened myself to the wonder of love, joy, and the creation of love. The night before my daughter's delivery, my husband bathed me in lavender and rose oil; we lit candles and said prayers. In the morning we laughed with delight all the way to the hospital. The doctors were smiling, the nurses were caring, and I finally appreciated the beauty of my daughter arriving into this world the way she wanted to come. As soon as I chose to experience the magic of love in a situation I initially felt was devastating, life unfolded for miracles and serendipities to take place. So much so that that my daughter arrived in perfect time to have an almost identical astrology to my husband. They both have Gemini in Sun, Mercury and Mars with a Leo ascendant. This is a testament to the divine universe always having a grander plan to what we could conjure up ourselves.

Another example could be waiting for the bus and getting increasingly bored. Every time you experience boredom, you are actually shutting yourself down and preventing love to interact with you. In such situations you could scan your environment and see what lights up to interact and exchange with you. It could be a tree, the person standing next to you, or some higher thought that sparks your mind with new awareness. Love can bring you wisdom, connection, and joy at any given moment—all you have to do is make the choice to relate to it.

Each wave of love that you allow yourself to meet—whether it is from your own awareness, the heavens, another person, or a living thing such as a tree, flower, or star—is capable of offering highly intelligent information and energy that can refresh, reshape, and rejuvenate your life. Through this conscious call to be made love to by the universe, the cosmic flower of your body is able to receive waves of beautiful love vibrations that ripple through your body, your cells, and to your core where the infinite vibration of love exists. Through the process you enable the love inside and outside of you to unite and make love with each other. Love makes love to you, and the energy it generates beautifies your body and blesses the life around you.

When you learn to orgasm with the divine universe in every micro-moment of daily life, the sound that comes from this embrace is OM, the vibrational sound that unifies all of life with the energy of love. The orgasmic OM is the divine universe making love to itself. And you, beautiful woman, are the divine universe in human form making love to all of life. Every cell in your body has the potential to OM and harmonize with all other OMs that have been vocalized from the beginning of time. OM is the sound the goddess sighs when all of life makes love to her.

This is a truly sensational alignment - everything in your infinite paradigm, is constantly being compounded to become a more refined version of love. Just as a diamond forms under pressure. Your being will continuously rebirth into a more elevated version of love - if it is put under pressure, to keep choosing the virtues of love to master your life. This is not a test, but a beautiful love affair. It encourages you to romance every aspect of your life until, everything in it becomes love. All you have to do is keep following the trail of love, keep choosing the virtues of love, and keep transcending that which inhibits it, so the magical moments of love can occur often . . . and always.

Reflection:

1. What does intimacy mean to you? What does it feel like to you?
2. Reflect upon your most intimate experiences. What words would you use to describe it?
3. What does it mean to gift your partner with your unique essence and vice versa?
4. What does consent mean to you? What does it mean to consent with your voice, your eyes, your body language, and your energy field?
5. Have you ever said yes when you actually meant no? Reflect upon your experiences. What would you tell your younger self?
6. How do consent and intimacy go hand in hand?
7. What does it mean to be unshakable with love?
8. List at least one hundred different ways that you can have a love affair with life.

13

Powerful, Magical Woman

The more you align every breath of your body and every moment of your life to love, the more powerful you will become. To be supported, guided, encouraged, inspired, and cherished by love is humanity's true spiritual quest. From love, peace follows and harmony flows, wisdom fortifies, and the courage of love transforms any obstacle. The power of love gives purpose and direction. Compassion melts barriers of racism, prejudice and inequality. Plus, the sheer joy and wonder of love blossoming everywhere in your life, offers continuous liberation from the mundane. You cannot exist without love, and so choosing to live with it, from it, and because of it, will challenge you to continuously awaken to the highest version of yourself—and the highest version of yourself is infinite, because love is infinite. Love is your superpower, helping you to master both yourself and life.

'Love is your superpower, helping you to master both yourself and life.'

Power for a woman who is aligned to love is not necessarily the traditional and masculine concept of power (achievement, progress, physical strength, comparison, superiority, and measurable financial resources). A woman's power is unable to be qualified or quantified; it is often invisible and always relies on a woman's ability to recognize her own personal power. True personal power will find you unshakable in the values of love and dynamic enough to use them to promote transformation in all areas of your life. No part of your life can be denied. Love gives you the tools to recognize your self-worth, the keys to master your relationships, the inspiration for your ambitions, and the conviction to attain them. Love helps you overcome obstacles, so you never feel defeated. It teaches that you always deserve to experience and create abundance. This is true power—not a need to dominate others or compete for resources, but rather a power that is ever evolving and eternal, benefitting all. This power is felt as a dynamic force throughout your entire body; it sings through your voice, dances off your hips, puts a spring in your step, and a knowing in your bones. It enlivens you instead of draining you. With this power, there is no stress or exhaustion because you are no longer striving for success; instead you are reconstructing your life to exist from love. Power for the enlightened woman is not a linear experience; it is multidimensional and can occur in every moment—from an awakening on the dance floor that changes the direction of your life, to requesting that your salary match your worth. True power promotes change that advances all—it's an enlightenment that moves beyond your own expansion to include those around you. Power is always granted to those who empower.

Eight Ways to Use Love as a Powerful Force of Transformation

1. The Power of Intuition

The power of intuition is a gift. It is often referred to as psychic abilities and commonly known as "women's intuition." Intuition is received through *clairvoyance*: clear seeing; *clairaudience*: clear hearing; *clairsentience*: clear feeling; and *prophetic sense*: clear knowing. For some, intuition can include visions or hearing messages, while others experience feelings, premonitions, or dreams. Whatever form intuition comes in, women have an uncanny ability to translate the messages being sent to them from the divine universe. Such messages have a profound impact upon your life, giving you insights into people, helping you navigate through problems, and providing you with direction and guidance to up-level your life to experience more love.

Love helps you see beyond your own paradigm. It teaches you to understand the truth of reality, from the perspective of the divine universe. It grants psychic depth, which means you are able to perceive the highest truth for yourself and others, plus a greater vision of the earth's and humanities evolution toward love. Love is not exclusive; it is inclusive to the greatest good of all. Psychic depth brings clarity and the foresight to develop all relationships and situations into something greater. This ability supports others to transform and evolve. Psychic depth brings assertive intuition to both manage and lead others. No longer will you collapse into doom, feel powerless to make a change, or feel obligated to enter into something you know is not right for you. Love always brings the truth, and coded deep within you is the knowing that you can change, transform, and heal any situation that crosses your path.

2. The Power to Transform

As you develop, it will become easier and easier to intuitively pick up clues from your environment that inspire you to transform and grow into a better version of yourself. To be able to elevate every aspect is power. To be able to transform your poverty consciousness into an abundance mindset is power. To be able to leave a relationship that is no longer working is power. To educate yourself so you can move to the next level of your career is power. You only need to follow the glow inside your body that is always whispering that you can be more, you can grow, you can transform.

3. The Power to Heal

You have the ability to channel and weave the healing energy of love into every you do. Your smile can bring another joy, the dinner you make can be medicine for those who eat it. The clothes you wash can become protection for those who wear them. Your words can sow peace and resolve arguments with ease. The love that emits from your being is healing. You are a walking portal of love, and you have the ability alleviate those whom you encounter.

4. The Power of Change

Since love is a dynamic force, your female energy is also meant to be fluid with the ability to dance with ever-changing life. The power to change enables the flexibility of when to start, when to stop, when to set boundaries, when to be assertive, when to be silent, when to talk, and when to confront. It teaches you when to celebrate, when to destroy, when to create, and when to be patient. Patience is a component of change, and it grants the time needed for all things to develop as intended, and so all will take place in the perfect time. Sometimes you will be required to focus on one action at a time, while other times you might use all these all actions at once. This dance of change is perfectly synchronized with the universe. You will feel, hear, and see what needs to happen before acting them out in physical reality. As a woman of love, you work together with the divine as a team, together co-creating heaven in your life through change. The more your life aligns to the greater truth, the easier it becomes for your magnificence to impact reality; the quicker the universe can reflect your brilliance back through physical manifestations. This can include your career, family, relationships, and the everyday experience of luxury and abundance.

5. The Power of Intention

A woman's belief is a very powerful thing. When you believe in a cause or a person, that very thing becomes both protected and supported by the love in the universe. As a woman, your belief is a life force, your intentions create protection, and your compassion activates a blessing. Every powerful woman knows she is the creator of her life. It is through intention and unwavering belief that your reality takes shape to support your desires. How else will you manifest your versions of love into physical reality?

6. The Power to Inspire

The power to inspire is the ability to bring life to both the self and others by believing in them, motivating them, and inspiring them to follow their dreams. Inspiration is a motivating force filled with wisdom, direction, encouragement, and guidance. It can flood your body with energy and desire, or whisper kind words to redirect your life. The more you inspire yourself, the more you will be able to inspire others, and the more the universe will inspire you. Love is an inspirational force, activating everything to keep blossoming into a better version.

7.   The Power to Speak

A voice is a beautiful thing, and a simple sound vibration can enter into the heart of whoever hears it. As you master love, you will learn to communicate without creating conflict or drama. You will discover how to use words that inspire, awaken, and create positive change in the listener. Of course, to speak means that you know how to listen, and to listen means that you are open to learning from others. Your words are powerful; they can create an alchemical change in your reality. They can unlock the mind of the listener to begin operating from love. Choose the right words and you will impact others, and therefore your life, in greater ways.

8.   The Power of Your Sexual Energy as a Sacred Life Force

The more you refine and align yourself to love, the more powerful your sexual energy will become, and the more you can use it as a sacred force of enlightenment in your life. As you become unshakable with the values of love internally, your body will naturally learn to tune into the experiences of love externally. From here you are able to both birth love and simultaneously become love. Your sexual energy then has no choice but to advance as a power that ignites a sense of strength and purpose from your genitals to your head. It expands as a feeling of sovereignty through your energy body and as a wave of transformation into your life. Your sexual energy is a powerhouse of energy, and when it joins forces with the vibration of love, it turns into an energy that can revolutionize every aspect of your life: your sense of worth, increasing your potential to experience heightened states pleasure, the confidence that helps you confront your partner to elevate their life so you can exchange more love, your ability to communicate diplomatically and disarm arguments, the certainty that you deserve to experience and create more abundance in your life, the sensations of intuitive guidance that ripple from the universe into your body, and the knowing that you have the ability to heal anything in your life that is out of alignment to love.

'Your sexual energy radiates from many places.'

Your sexual power radiates from many places and awakens you to stand stronger, act more boldly, and live more vibrantly. As it sublimates to become a sacred source of energy, it will bring life to your cells, words to your mouth, movement to your muscles, passion to your heart, and purpose to your mind. It is a creative force that can shift the molecules of reality to behave in new ways and awaken your manifestations into physical reality. Your sexual power is a catalyst and a remedy that progresses on your spiritual path. You cannot master yourself in this world without it. It is an integral part of your human existence and an essential component to every awakening you have into love. Your sexual energy is the sacred key that will unlock your health, your vibrancy, your confidence, your self-worth and self-love, your intimacy in relationships, and your luck in life. A woman who suppresses her sexual energy remains lifeless and disconnected from the embodiment of love. But a woman who chooses to cultivate her sacred sexual energy ignites both her body and her life to experience the divinity in everything—and divinity in the physical world is a very sensual, enlightening experience. You, beautiful woman, live in the most exquisite body, one that is powerful beyond measure. You live because your sexual energy desires to experience the freedom of love.

Exercise: Transforming Your Life with the Power of Your Sacred Energy - *refer to figure 13:*

1. Stand tall with your feet hip-distance apart. Begin this meditation by swaying and moving your hips to awaken your sexual energy. You may also want to charge your sexual energy with the earth's energy. Or, stretch your hands to the sky to charge your body with sunlight, starlight and heavenly energy.
2. Allow your sexual energy the freedom to move through your body with the blossoming techniques in Chapter 6. The focus is to let your sexual energy ignite the love within, until it glows from your skin. This should start to make you feel both vibrant and strong in your body.
3. Now visualize the vibration of love that exists all around you and inhale it into all the cells of your body. As you do, intend it to ignite your sexual energy even more. Exhale and breathe out the

radiant energy through all of your cells. Repeat until your energy/auric body begins to glow. This should make you feel stronger and in command of life.

4. Keep allowing your body to blossom with your sexual energy and the vibration of love. You can use any of the body blossoming techniques in chapter six to facilitate this. The key is to keep expanding your energy through your body and out into life. Expand it to include your relationships, your workplace, your home, and even the entire planet. This should make you feel deeply intimate and in command of all of life.

5. From the depths of your being, where the purest part of your essence resides, make an intention for what you would like to create or manifest in your life. Exhale and breathe that intention through all of your cells, letting it encode the love within you and your sexual energy with new information. Witness this new vibration of energy shining from your being. Recoding the molecules of reality to behave in new ways supportive to your manifestation. In this moment, you may feel the energy of new opportunities arriving, or the people that no longer support you leaving. You may also get inspired to take actions that activate your manifestations into physical reality.

6. Finally, stand with your palms open to receive and your heart awakened with gratitude. Welcome your manifestation into your life. Notice the molecules in your body shifting to align with it.

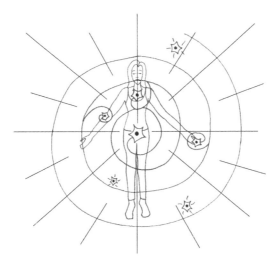

Figure 13: Transforming Your Life With Your Sacred Energy

Reflection:

1. What does *power* mean to you?
2. How would you describe yourself as a powerful and magical woman?
3. Of the eight ways to use love as a powerful force, which do you find the easiest to do?
4. Which do you find the hardest to do? Why? What can you do to help this?
5. What does "sublimate your sexual energy into a sacred life force" mean to you?
6. What areas of your life need to be transformed?
7. How can your energy field positively impact your reality?
8. How can you allow the universe to help you more?
9. What is your greatest heart desire right now?

14

You Are A Sacred Woman & Your Love Is Revolutionary

*E*very woman is a sacred vessel who has the ability to birth into existence many types of creations. Every woman is inherently intuitive and gifted with many talents. Your quest is to realize your authentic self and radiate your unique expression into life. This journey begins once you accept yourself as sacred.

No man, no person, no teaching, or teacher can activate your divinity—only you can. You must claim your beauty, your wisdom, your creativity, your intuition, and your sexuality as precious. Once you invoke this rite of passage, you become a goddess, a sacred woman, a sensual yogini.

As you awaken, there is a deep yearning to be loved, appreciated, respected, and honored. This desire is sent as a call from the depths of your heart into the universe. You ask for life to resynchronize and align to your magnificence. You long to radiate your unique authentic self, and the divine universe longs to reflect your brilliance.

Relationships and opportunities will become more abundant as you

203

recognize that you are supported and cared for. This will allow you to relax, surrender, and open yourself to more blessings, more miracles, more sensuality, more pleasure, and more aliveness in your body. You have the ability to feel appreciated, satisfied, and ignited by all of creation.

In response to this awakening, gratitude will pour from your heart into the infinite universe. You will shine with so much love that it fuels your physical body and ignites your sexual energy to expand into the higher realms of your magnificence. As you align to your unique truth and merge with life, you become wedded to all that is. This union is sacred and grants you the power to create. Manifesting your version of heaven on earth will become your only occupation.

Through this process, you will learn to trust that every experience you encounter is an opportunity to embrace the infinite ways love can express itself into reality. You desire to manifest more bliss in your life, and you require the gifts of intuition and healing to accomplish this. Just as a lotus flower emerges from the mud before it can blossom, you will begin to understand that certain things in your life act like the mud and must be transcended. Your keen intuition allows you to spot all that remains lacking, and your healing abilities transform them into abundance. Relationships move out of conflict and become effortless. Opportunities stop being unattainable and become available. As you weed your garden of the unwanted, you will reseed it with all that aligns to your brilliance. You will die and rebirth yourself a million times until perfection is reached. You are psychic and always one with the mystery and source of all that is. Never alone, you commune with everything.

The most luxurious communion you will have is with your body. Wild and succulent, tender and beautiful, fearless and free, your deliciousness has no boundaries. The more you dive into self-love, the more you can cherish your body as a temple. The temple that houses the goddess is a holy space, and everything within it is sacred. Every thought, emotion, experience, inspiration, and sensation are honored as divine. Life and passion are released from your cells, and you will continuously discover yourself as both powerful and sensual. You, beautiful woman, will become alive with life and continuously command more love to abide within and around you. Your feminine soul always requests to be deeply nourished. And so it is.

The end is always the beginning...
Continue your journey and enjoy your free gift here:
www.vanyasilverten.com/sensual

About The Author

Vanya Silverten works internationally as an intuitive energy healer and teacher. With clients and students from over 50 countries, she has a passion to help individuals transform all aspects of their lives. Her greatest joy is to teach people the skills of healing and intuition so that they can master their own lives. Vanya believes healing is an art, and so has refined her gifted intuition through the experience of treating, reading and teaching 10,000+ people. She has developed the energetic understanding of how the body, mind and soul functions through her extensive training and experience. She passes this knowledge on by teaching and qualifying students to become practitioners of Theta Healing®

In 2015, Vanya became a mother to a beautiful daughter. This life changing experience has deepened her appreciation of the exquisite female body temple and its potential to reach heighten states of sensual enlightenment. You can learn how to unlock the sensual magic of your body with her retreats and online trainings. For more details go to www. vanysilverten.com

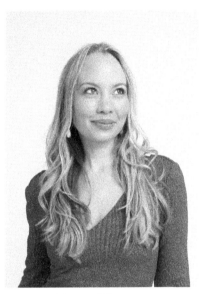

Vanya Silverten

**'May this book become a gift you give to your sisters,
daughters, friends, and any woman who is in need of love.'**

About The Artist

Leona Matuszak is a Visual Artist and Lead Art Workshop Facilitator based in London, U.K. Leona feels that the process of making art is important for both personal development and bringing people together from all backgrounds and cultures. She graduated with a degree in Applied Arts in 2001 and has numerous sculptural and mosaic public artworks located across London. Leona created *Artists Resource* in 2011 with the Mission "To bring people together to nurture Creativity and facilitate Transformation – for the benefit of the individual and the community." Explore her unique art classes and online courses here: www.artistsresource.co.uk

Lightning Source UK Ltd.
Milton Keynes UK
UKHW041504080620
364652UK00002B/515